RIDE
TO LIFE

Dr Gary M. Leong
MB BS FRACP PhD

First published 2020 by Gary M. Leong
This edition published 2022

Produced by Indie Experts P/L, Australasia
indieexperts.com.au

Copyright © Gary M. Leong 2020

The moral right of the author to be identified as the author of this work has been asserted.

All rights reserved. Except as permitted under the *Australian Copyright Act 1968*, no part of this publication may be reproduced, stored in a retrieval system, or transmitted in any form or by any means, electronic, mechanical, photocopying, recording or otherwise, without prior written permission from the publisher. All enquiries should be made to the author.

Cover design by Maria Biaggini
Edited by Samantha Sainsbury
Internal design by Indie Experts
Typeset by Post Pre-press Group, Brisbane

ISBN 978-0-6486712-5-1 (hardback)
ISBN 978-0-6486712-4-4 (paperback)
ISBN 978-0-6486712-6-8 (epub)

Disclaimer:
We advise that the information contained in this book does not negate personal responsibility on the part of the reader for their own health and safety. It is recommended that individually tailored advice is sought from your healthcare or medical professional. The publishers and their respective employees, agents and authors, are not liable for injuries or damage occasioned to any person as a result of reading or following the information contained in this book.

RIDE
TO LIFE

A no-nonsense program for breaking your family's cycle of obesity and diabetes for a healthier, happier thriving life

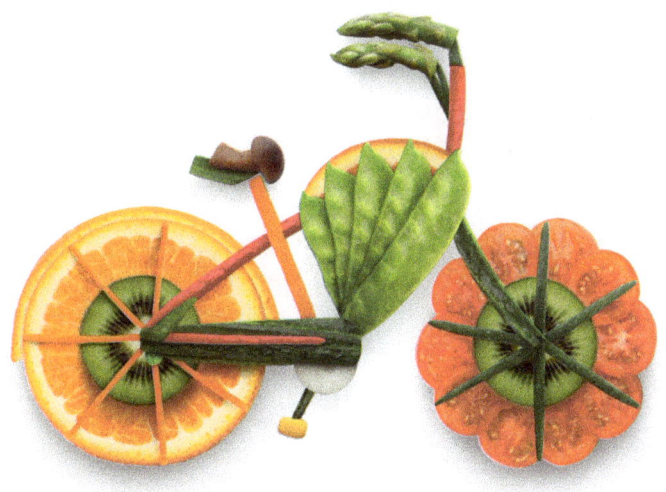

Dr Gary M. Leong
MB BS FRACP PhD

Contents

Foreword	vii
Introduction	1
A story to inspire your family	4
Background on obesity	7
Tackling the issue	12
How to read this book and work through the program	15

PARTIE 1 – GET ON YOUR BIKE!

Taking responsibility for where you are now — 21

Stage 1 – Get honest: understanding where you are and why	23
Stage 2 – Decision time: committing to a healthier life	37
Stage 3 – Getting ready for change: preparing for the ride to a connected life	47

PARTIE 2 – IN TRAINING

What it takes to break the obesity cycle for your family — 77

Stage 4 – Go within: why reclaiming life starts with mindfulness	79
Stage 5 – You are what you eat: nutrition for making the change for good	97
Stage 6 – Get moving! Learning to love exercise and move your body consciously!	121
Stage 7 – Sleep, Problematic Internet Use (PIU) and its effects on cognitive function and mental and physical health	147

PARTIE 3 – ON THE ROAD

In training and doing the hard yards — 155

Stage 8 – Connection, self-care and support — 157

Stage 9 – The power of 'no': why you need it and how to use it. — 169

Stage 10 – Body image, self-esteem and communication — 179

Stage 11 – Setbacks and relapses: why they happen and how to get back on the bike — 185

PARTIE 4 – MAINTAIN AND SUSTAIN

Staying on the bike even after the main event — 195

Stage 12 – The future's bright: dreaming big and creating a new reality — 197

Stage 13 – Connect and care: why community helps and how it pays to be part of one — 203

Stage 14 – The final stage on your Champs-Élysées! — 209

Acknowledgements — 211

About Dr Gary Leong — 213

Speaking opportunities — 215

Endnotes — 217

Foreword

Gary or Dr K, or Dr Koala, as some call him, is no ordinary children's doctor! Over the last four years, I have had the pleasure of riding with Dr K on several major Smiling for Smiddy (SFS) five-day cycle challenges to raise money for cancer research for the Mater Foundation Brisbane. Along with Mark 'Sharky' Smoothy, the founder of SFS, we have ridden together during cycle challenges around Noosa in Queensland, New Zealand's South Island and most recently in Tasmania.

Dr K has a passion and commitment to being physically active with his cycling. He uses this in part to inspire the families and children he sees in his clinic who suffer from obesity and diabetes. He, in turn, is inspired by the amazing people within and outside the Smiddy peloton, including his fellow riders and all the many health professionals he has worked with in Australia and overseas.

But he gains most inspiration from the many families he has the privilege to care for in his clinics in Brisbane and Sydney. These families come to him for advice about their children on how best to manage and improve their severe obesity and its many serious ill-effects on mental and physical health.

In this book, Dr K has poured his 30 years of training and acquired wisdom into developing a program to inspire and transform the lives of children and their families suffering from obesity. It emphasises the importance of a whole-of-family-based approach, including healthy nutrition and being physically active outdoors, either by riding your bicycle, walking, swimming or taking part in any enjoyable physical activity and movement that allows you to experience beautiful natural places and new adventures together as a family.

As a former pro-cyclist and now 'Senior Ambassador' of Australian cycling, I can attest to the enormous beneficial effects of outdoor physical activity on my health and wellbeing, and in the prevention of obesity, diabetes and mental illness in the community.

I wish Dr K all the best with his new book and the Ride to Life program to inspire more families to start an active, healthy life.

Mr Phil Anderson OAM of Phil Anderson Cycling

In 1981, Phil was the first Australian, and in fact the first non-European, pro-cyclist to wear the maillot jaune (yellow jersey), which is awarded to the leader of Le Tour de France professional cycle race. He also wore the maillot jaune during the 1982 Tour de France.

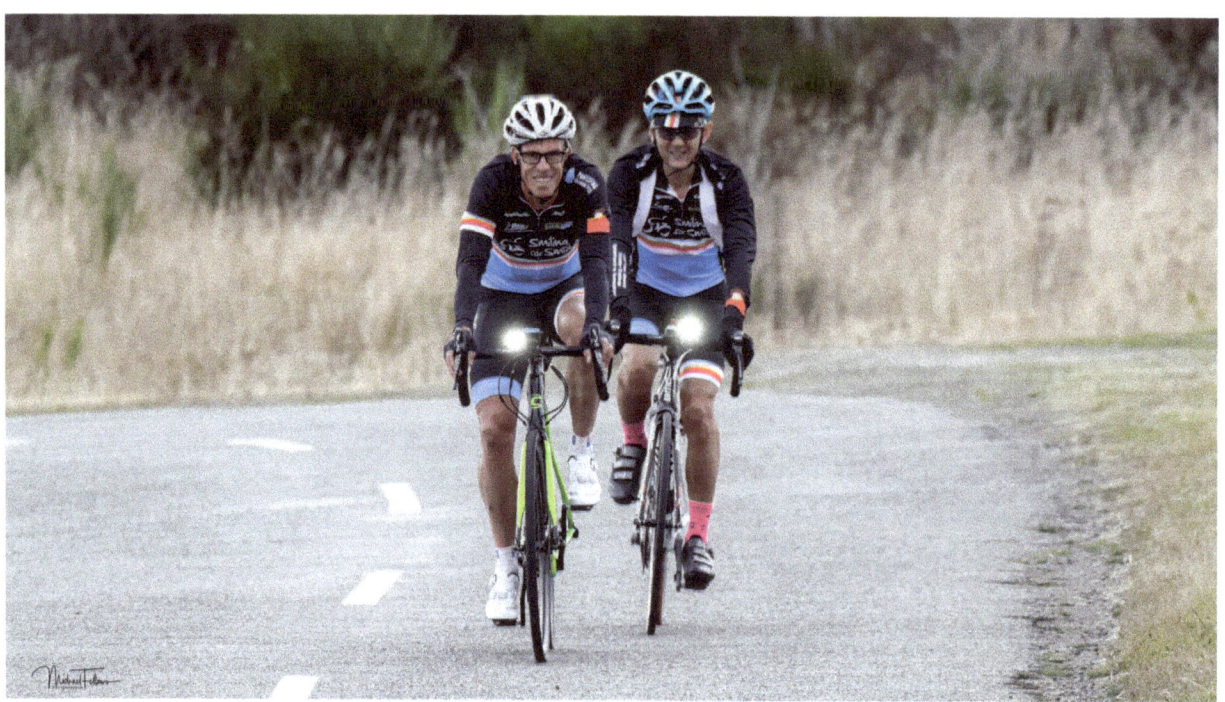

Phil 'Skippy' Anderson riding with Dr.Koala in Christchurch on 2017 New Zealand Smiddy Challenge.
Image courtesy of Michael Fellows and the Mater Foundation.

Introduction

Your journey starts here

I am a paediatrician (a children's doctor), and a paediatric endocrinologist (a doctor qualified to diagnose and treat disorders of the endocrine glands and hormones in children). But most importantly I am a father of three children (now all adults) and in many ways I have learnt more about childhood and its problems through bringing up my own children with my caring wife than from any textbook of paediatrics!

Through my clinical practice I have treated hundreds of children and families at public and private clinics in Sydney and Brisbane, including at the KOALA clinic and the Kids Fit 4 Future Clinic.

When these children and their families come to see me, the whole family is often overwhelmed and at a loss as to how to address the terrible health condition of obesity afflicting their child. They often feel guilty, ashamed, demoralised, stuck, disconnected, mired in negativity and sometimes desperate.

Over many years working closely with these families, I sensed and then knew – there was more to obesity as a condition, or disease as some experts advocate it be designated. It wasn't just purely a medical condition due to excessive fat accumulation in the body leading to an unhealthy increase in weight. And this meant it couldn't just be treated with purely medical solutions. We have heard it all before, haven't we? Just eat less and move more and you will be fine. Well, for most overweight and obese children and adults, this is easier said than done, as the body becomes both accustomed in a way, as it were, to this increase in body weight and any effort to try to lose weight is counteracted by strong involuntary hormonal forces that protects against any weight loss achieved through lifestyle changes. While this has been well documented now in several rigorous clinical research studies, the other just as powerful force preventing many children and their families from staying a healthy weight is, in my opinion, related to psychosocial and socio-cultural factors. Many of these are ingrained in the parents during their own upbringing and subsequently influence their own children's behaviour, but more about that later.

Thus, it has become apparent to me that there are many unseen aspects to obesity. There are mental, emotional and social elements to the condition that aren't really addressed by mainstream medicine. As a paediatrician, this was a big issue for me to think about and try to address. How could I best help my patients and their parents?

While I was trained to diagnose and treat children medically, after years of practice I felt this approach was only working to a point. Increasingly, I felt I was not doing the best by my patients and their parents just looking at things in a purely medical context. I felt compelled to bring a more integrated approach to treatment. I found the emotional, mental and socio-cultural aspects of the disease must be considered equally too.

This book outlines a potentially life-changing program that I have developed called the Ride to Life program. It encourages you to courageously and honestly confront the underlying reasons for the obesity affecting your child. But it is also about parents *and* children taking appropriate levels of personal responsibility *and* then taking action to make sustainable, manageable change for a better, healthier, active and more purposeful life. This book attempts to solve the problem about what you can do as a parent when you think you have run out of options for a child suffering from obesity.

Having said that, right up front I want to state that this book offers no quick fixes. Nor does it offer rocket science, a fad diet, or a silver bullet. If you think your child's current health challenges will be solved this way, this is not the book or program for you. In fact, if you are looking for a quick solution, I do not think you will find any book or program anywhere that will help you. You and your family have to do the work and then your child will become empowered by your effort and start to thrive.

It's easy to get stuck when we feel overwhelmed by a situation that feels too hard. Old habits, limiting beliefs and negative thinking creep in and take hold, preventing us from progressing towards our dreams. At times, we even lose sight of what's most important in our lives and we neglect what we value most in our own health and our family's health.

One reason I wrote this book is because of my own experience of disconnection. For many years I was heavily focused on work. I neglected other important areas of my life – the mental, emotional, social and spiritual. In short, I became 'disconnected'. Having treated hundreds of patients suffering with obesity, I've observed this is how they often feel too. A timely, serious bike accident caused me to pause, reflect, change and take better self-care. Unfortunately, often a catastrophic event is required before we'll take action. I've found many parents in my clinics have had the same experience; it's just their challenge is addressing the underlying reasons for the obesity and its adverse effects on every aspect of their child's life.

But remarkable change is possible for those who are courageous enough to make a decision, get honest, accept personal responsibility and enact change. Through this book you and your child can proudly own and cherish your responsibility and make lasting change for good.

I've seen despairing families on the brink of collapse turn things around with the help of the principles and advice outlined in this book. I wish you very possible success and you know you have my and my team's support. You've taken the first step in buying this book. The power is in your hands. I wish you every possible success.

Dr Gary 'Koala' Leong

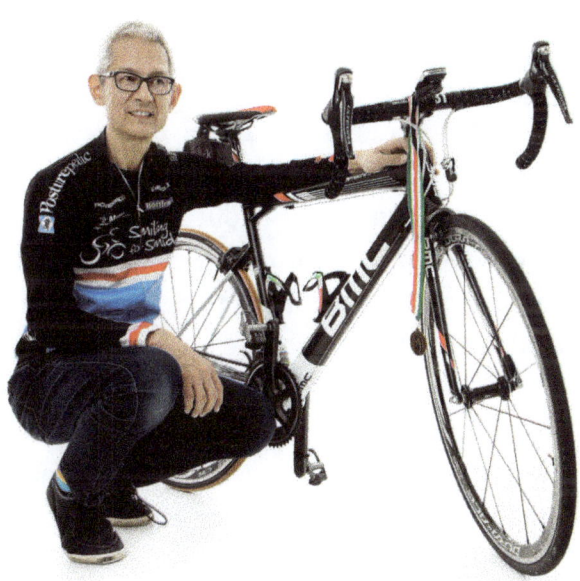

A story to inspire your family

I first met Charlie when he and his mother arrived at my clinic for help with his obesity and major behaviour problems. At age six he already weighed 55kg with a BMI of almost 33kg/m^2, which put him in the extreme obesity range. Charlie was born weighing 5kg and with diabetic macrosomia, and was always hungry from day one. He consumed large amounts of milk in infancy, and unhealthy and processed foods became a mainstay in his diet as he developed. Many of Charlie's behavioural issues were governed by his continuous desire to eat processed foods and snacks.

His mother had pre-diabetes and through her pregnancies had severe insulin-dependent gestational diabetes. Her most recent pregnancy inspired her to diet and exercise to lose 40kg in three years. However, her family were not greatly supportive of her efforts to change the family food environment, and her husband, though caring, was not concerned about his children's unhealthy eating and excessive weight. Through much determination and against most of her family's expressed will, she managed to make some significant changes to her children's nutrition and physical activity levels, learning how to stay strong when Charlie and his siblings nagged her for unhealthy food.

With these changes, Charlie's weight stabilised as he grew so that by seven-and-a-half years of age and still weighing 55 kg, but having grown taller, his BMI had fallen to just below 30kg/m^2. While this was still well above an optimal healthy weight range, it was an amazing achievement.

A bonus outcome for Charlie was that, although he had been diagnosed with autism and attention-deficit-hyperactivity disorder (ADHD), with healthy fresh food and regular daily physical activity his behaviour, and that of his brother too, improved enormously. His school grades, learning aptitude and sleep patterns also improved remarkably, further emphasising the impact of nutritious foods and movement on brain chemistry. Charlie has a natural desire to move and eat healthily now, and does not feel continuously hungry.

With continued vigilance and determination for her family's long-term health, Charlie's mother is a true inspiration for her own family as well as many others facing severe obesity and the risk of chronic disease.

A true and inspiring story of MOTHER POWER!

I think this journey with my kids is the hardest, and most trying thing I have ever done.

Having to motivate myself and change my own ways as a woman, and as a mother and role model is the most challenging. While it is truly a daily struggle, it is also very rewarding at the same time

My kids are my world. Charlie, James and Anton are everything I could ever want and more, and although they all come with their individual battles, they are my personal inspiration to become better. I know that by my efforts to better myself, one day all my hard work will pay off.

Charlie's heart is bigger than life. He has a great love for food, and for life. Like many kids, he has to fight for acceptance, and struggles with making the right choices about food or his behaviour. But he has an unending drive to never fail, and to always try his best, no matter the outcome. I know he always trusts that I have his best interests at heart.

Charlie's long journey with food and his addiction to it has been super hard and trying at times, but what an achievement that he has now become able to manage his weight. Although still overweight for his age, he has maintained his strict schedule of exercise and eating regimen for 3 years. Although I do the cooking and preparing, he is the one who has done it. I have just pushed him along the way now.

I find it to be inspirational he has learned to overcome his own daily battles of being bullied and teased. To me he is an eight year old champion and one day he will come to the realisation that he did this. He put in the hard work and he will continue to do so going forward, with a more positive attitude and relationship with food. Whatever I have asked of him, he does, and he does it with all his heart.

Being healthy is huge in my house. Does one size fit all? NO WAY! Is it a lot of trial and error? YES! 100 percent. What works for one kid, sure as hell doesn't work for all of them, but I've learned that being healthy is not just about the way you look or what a set of scales reads. I have come to believe a healthy gut means you will have a healthy mind, and a healthy mind means you will have a healthy life.

More, more, and more food is not the answer, and less, less, and less is not either. It's finding a happy medium. A balance of a little bit of everything in moderation. That is the answer and it really is as simple as that.

In all honesty I use to be 146 kilos which I know was huge! I now weigh 84 kilos, and my own lifestyle and battles were insane. I was a diabetic on daily insulin, plus tablets. Having a heart attack at 33 years of age put me on my arse quicker than anything. My high cholesterol, high blood pressure, diabetes and my life loaded with stress. This was not ideal!

Every day, I now make a conscious decision as to whether I am going to live for myself and my children, or whether I'm going to die. And I choose every day to LIVE. I choose to be here for those three boys. That's what gets me up every morning. As their mother I will do all I can to forever make good choices in our diet and lifestyle. We try our hardest to be better and healthier versions of ourselves. I decided I want to live a long life, as I want the same thing for my kids too.

I don't have any extra support. It's me and them all the way. So, I know I need to make sure that they all have the correct information, the right life skills. I need to make sure that they will be ready for this harsh world we all live in. Having autism and ADHD and so many other things is hard.

Food plays a huge role in life, and they will need all their own tools to be ready in that tool box for when I'm not around. To make sure that they are set up for life, and no matter what, they will be ready to take on the world. This also means they will be ready to pass on what I have taught them to the people they meet, and eventually onto their own kids.

It comes down to this: this journey that we have all been on, is so much more than dieting and exercise; it's about making a choice to live. That choice is called a healthy lifestyle change.

Background on obesity

Obesity: it's more than physical

When we look at obesity as a purely physical condition, we miss so much of what is required to live, be healthier and have a more fulfilled, purposeful life. We make recovery harder and we disregard the importance of the many other aspects of this condition that must be addressed if we're to create lasting solutions and healthier, happier lives for our kids. It's why I tell people recovery from obesity starts on the inside by addressing mental and emotional aspects of the condition. For me, treating obesity is an 'inside job' and it starts with you as the parents.

Now, I know that statement may upset a few people – including parents and a few of my medical peers. But my experience and research points to the need for a novel approach that takes into account the psychosocial and cultural context of the whole family. That is, the daily lives of each individual family member and the connection – or lack of it – between them and their extended community.

Imagine your child is sitting in the middle of a web, connected to a greater or lesser extent to all other family members – parents, siblings, grandparents and the extended family. Then consider the connections to community, school, church or sporting club. Of course, our connections go well beyond the few I've mentioned; however, the impact of a small movement – a change in behaviour – can be felt by all who are connected to the web. Some may support change, while others may resist. If your child is one caught in the web of obesity, change is necessary to create a healthier, happier life. It's essential for breaking the cycle that created the web of obesity in the first place.

It's my belief that the emergence of obesity in children is nearly always the result of inter-generational emotional, mental and social issues that haven't been addressed in the parents and even in the grandparents perhaps, often around their own childhood and adolescence. As unpalatable as this may be, the flipside is: managing and recovering from obesity is in the hands of the parents and children who are most affected. We just need to learn how to take personal responsibility, while discarding past mistakes and associated guilt to embrace a healthier future. My experience as a paediatrician tells me this is the most sustainable and effective way to recovery. Research shows obesity is linked to social disadvantage, reflected in a lack of education and opportunities. This lack of education has to be overcome but that is what the Ride to Life program will help you and your family do.

Obesity: the global health crisis

The global obesity epidemic, and it is an epidemic, has crept up on us. In 2022, the reality is that one in every four Australian children is either overweight or obese. Childhood obesity is one of the biggest challenges facing this generation of children and the planet as a whole. Now prevalent in all Western countries and a growing number of second and third world countries,[1] the explosion in the number of overweight people and people with obesity has caused specialists to look at the disease differently.

World Health Organization key facts

- In 2016, more than 1.9 billion adults, 18 years and older, were overweight (52% of all adults). Of these over 650 million were obese (13%).
- Most of the world's population lives in countries where being overweight and obesity kills more people than being underweight.
- In 2016, 41 million children under the age of five, and over 340 million children and adolescents aged five–19, were overweight or obese.
- Overweight and Obesity are major risk factors for Type 2 Diabetes mellitus (T2DM) and Heart Disease. Both these diseases are preventable though a healthy active lifestyle.
- Heart Disease which includes coronary artery disease, heart arrhythmia and heart failure, is still the leading cause of death in both men and women.
- Obesity also increases the risk of high blood pressure and stroke, obstructive sleep apnoea, mental illness, dementia and Alzheimer's disease, fatty liver disease, various musculoskeletal conditions and several common cancers, such as breast, pancreas, oesophagus, bowel, kidney and liver cancer. Thus children, adolescents and adults who suffer from obesity have higher rates of these chronic diseases and of premature death.

- In 2021, according to the International Diabetes Federation (IDF) Diabetes Atlas (10th Edition), there were 537 million people living with diabetes (90% have T2DM) or 1 in 10 people. Another 541 million people have pre-diabetes in the world.
- The number of people with diabetes globally is alarmingly predicted to increase to 643 million in 2030 and 784 million in 2045, a 45 % increase.
- This has led the IDF to state 'Diabetes is the fastest growing global health emergency of the 21st century', costing globally almost 1 trillion USD annually.
- While the unpreventable form of diabetes, Type 1 Diabetes mellitus (T1DM) remains the main type of diabetes in children, the prevalence of children and adolescents with overweight and obesity with T2DM is rising.
- Those youth at greatest risk of T2DM arise from indigenous populations around the globe, including our Aboriginal and Torres Strait Islanders, New Zealand Maori and South Pacific Islanders, as well as African-Americans, South-East Asia including China, India and Pakistan, the Middle East, and Hispanic populations in all parts of the Americas.
- Youth with T2DM are at much greater risk of diabetes complications (including eye, kidney and liver and nervous system) than youth with T1DM.

There is now an emerging understanding that obesity is a function of globalisation, industrialisation, urbanisation, environmental change and economic development as much as anything else that contributes to the condition.[2] In her book, *The Big Fat Conspiracy*, Melissa Sweet suggests we cannot view obesity simplistically – a result of simply eating too much and not doing enough physical activity. Instead, we can see it as the consequence of a perfect storm of environmental factors arising from urbanisation and economic prosperity.[3] I would add to these factors the unaddressed social, mental and emotional issues, which sit underneath these issues and emerge as a result of the disconnection factors mentioned above.

So widely acknowledged is this epidemic that, in some circles, the term 'globesity' has been coined to describe what's really going on. It's enough to say generally, waistlines around the world are getting wider, and it's affecting our kids to the point where their lives and long-term health are threatened. I wouldn't be the first person to point out we're now dealing with a generation of children with obesity who are at risk of dying before their parents. I liken this phenomenon to a tsunami. Rising up, seemingly out of the blue, it has the potential to wreak incredible havoc and destruction. We ignore the problem at the peril of our kids' lives. And to a large degree, as parents, we must wear some of the responsibility, but also as parents we must recognise that we have the power to change this scenario in our family for the better.

For many families, the obesity 'tsunami' is reaching its peak in the current generation. In the USA where the child obesity epidemic has really hit hard, between 2002 and 2012 annual increases show that youths aged 10 to 19 years presenting with type 2 diabetes are now almost three times that of type 1 diabetes, the more common autoimmune-mediated and non-obesity-related form of childhood diabetes.[4] Thus the seeds for young adult heart disease are probably already sewn, given heart attack remains the major cause of death in adult men and women who were obese as adolescents.[5]

Don't think Australian children with obesity are not at significant risk of type 2 diabetes compared to their USA counterparts. With our multicultural society many ethnic populations are statistically at high risk of obesity-related type 2 diabetes. Sadly, this includes our own Indigenous population, but also includes large numbers of children from the South-Pacific and Maori ethnic background, central Asian including Indian and Pakistani ethnicity, and Chinese and Middle Eastern including Lebanese and Turkish ethnicities, who make up many of the beautiful families that I see in my clinics every week.

I am trying to say that these ethnic groups all have one thing in common – culturally they are food lovers with food used as an expression of love. Food, quantities and portion sizes have exploded and traditional healthier diets and lifestyles abandoned with adoption of Western-style, high-saturated fat, sugary diets and physically inactive sedentary lifestyles.

Many children I see in my clinic often have parents and grandparents living with obesity too. The fact is these parents and grandparents perhaps feel it's a function of ageing, and therefore are less motivated to change their course. What we're observing now is the onset of obesity is occurring much earlier than it ever did. Children now present with severe obesity as infants and toddlers. It's a demonstration that the condition is progressive, worsening and all too common.

One in seven Australian adults has diabetes, and this number only reflects the people who are aware they have diabetes. A more realistic figure is probably one in five. Over time, I've witnessed a progressive increase in the number of children I see who have obesity combined with severe insulin resistance, a precursor to pre-diabetes or type 2 diabetes mellitus (T2DM).

In addition, childhood obesity is now the major cause of fatty liver disease and contributes to the development of obstructive sleep apnoea. A generation ago, this was unheard of; now it is widely accepted. It's a sad fact that our children are suffering with adult diseases, which will inevitably reduce their quality of life and life expectancy if the underlying causes of their ill-health are not addressed.

Tackling the issue

The good news is, as a parent, you have enormous power in your hands, particularly if you're the mother. This is not to let the father, grandparents, or any other adult carer off the hook from responsibility! But the reality is, because they're often in the role of primary carers, it's mums who take the first steps to address obesity. It's not that dads, grandparents and carers aren't as important; they are. It's just that through my clinical experience I've found mums are:

- Often the primary caregiver in the family
- Often decision-makers on what food to buy and meals to prepare
- Usually the family cook and supervise meal times
- Frequently the ones who bring children to appointments
- Often the initiators of change
- Most commonly the first to seek help for their children when it's needed
- Often under estimate their power to influence their family
- Usually the first to blame themselves for the circumstances of their child's health concerns
- The people who are prepared to hold firm to new boundaries and behaviours, even in the face of criticism and pressure often unfortunately from their spouse or in-laws.

I also find mothers are most open to listening. Often, they are facing their own battle with obesity and want to help their child avoid the same issues they have experienced. Maybe you've struggled with your own health and wellbeing and are now staring down the barrel of having a child or children who also reflect the same struggle. Called to action by your child's health, you've decided enough is enough. My tip to you is: keep going.

I frequently see grandparents, and carers too, who have been left or forced to pick up the 'broken' pieces. Many families are confused about the increasing health issues associated with poor diet, a sedentary lifestyle and too much technology. They are searching for practical tools that work and can be implemented in everyday life.

Sometimes I see partners who know meaningful change is necessary if their family is to have any chance at enjoying a healthy future together. It is confusing for these people because they're unsure of how to approach the topic with their partner. Notwithstanding the importance of mums, the most effective approach is one that brings *both* parents along, working together. Where both parents are connected, proactive and supporting one another to break the cycle of obesity, there is greater chance of long-term, sustainable success. An important philosophy I repeat many times in this book is: 'One rule for all and all for one.'

How this book is written

One thing you should know about me is that I love to ride my bicycle. I am a dedicated and enthusiastic cyclist and have travelled the world with friends and family searching for new adventures and mountains to climb. I just love the challenge of cycling in beautiful, natural places and being connected to the positively inspiring people riding with me or supporting me.

For your healthier journey as a parent of a child with obesity you need to find the same connection to positively inspiring people and places to keep you going on your recovery. I see the challenge of deciding, preparing, training, doing the exercises described in this book and breaking the cycle of obesity as similar to endurance rides.

There are many times during the process of these long, arduous rides – from committing to the ride and physically completing it – where I faced my own resistance and challenges. Sometimes I didn't want to keep going. At times, I felt emotional, even weak. And I know the other riders did too. What compelled me to 'get back (and stay) on my bike' each time was the desire to keep myself healthy and emotionally well – and to serve others. And that desire keeps me going today.

In the same way, addressing the obesity issues facing your child and your family is like taking an endurance ride for life. There will be times when you want to give up and other times when it's plain sailing. The main goal though is to keep going, no matter what. Throughout the book, we talk about a positive growth mindset and it's critical you adopt this long-term mindset. There is no quick fix to your challenge. Remember it has taken a long time to reach this point; in some cases, it's taken generations. It's absolutely vital you remember that if you don't start, you won't get far along the ride to reverse your family's cycle of obesity. The ideas in this book apply to you, the parent, as much as they do to your child living with obesity. They also apply to every member of your family.

Earlier I said *Ride to Life* solves the problem about what to do when you feel like you're out of options. It does this in a non-judgemental and balanced way, which demonstrates empathy, but doesn't let people off the hook either. For things to change in a positive, sustainable way, each of us needs to take responsibility for our part. This includes children too. You will see throughout the book, there are references to children taking on age-appropriate responsibility for their health and wellbeing. There are also recommendations for you as a parent to allow your child to develop this resilience and take on the responsibility. This is an essential step, and sometimes a challenging one for parents; however, it's part of recovery and cannot be bypassed if your children are to enjoy a healthier, happier life.

I encourage you to think about the recovery of your child's health and restoration of balance in your and their life as the most important ride you'll ever take. Far more than a sprint, this will be an endurance ride that tests your mental and emotional resilience and physical strength, but one that will empower you and sustain you too.

How to read this book and work through the program

Ride to Life is a program and workbook. Written in four distinct parts or sections with bite-sized stages, you will see there are exercises throughout designed to make you think and take action.

La partie is the French word for the part, so use it also as reason to 'party' i.e. celebrate your progress from one section to the next with a healthy reward for the whole family.

Partie 1 – Get on your bike! Taking responsibility for where you are now
In Partie 1 we establish where you, your child and family are right now in terms of tackling obesity. Remember, no judgement. We must know our starting point before commencing the ride to a healthier life.

Partie 2 – In training: What it takes to break the obesity cycle for your family
We look at the key areas of life in which change needs to occur to break the cycle of obesity. While we look at the nutritional and physical aspects of change, we also address the mental/emotional aspects as well and how to involve your whole family.

Partie 3 – On the road: In training and doing the hard yards
A bit like training for a big ride, in this partie the rubber hits the road. Partie 3 is about implementation: putting things in place to bring about the necessary changes for a healthier, happier active and purposeful life for you and your child.

Partie 4 – Maintain and sustain: Staying on the bike even after the main event
Partie 4 is dedicated to keeping you on track. It can be easy to deviate from course when we're tired, overwhelmed and not feeling good. In this section, we look at tools for staying on your bike and continuing your Ride to Life.

As you read the book, I encourage you to be diligent. Read the stages carefully, do the exercises, check out the references and resources. Working this program *will* make a difference. You can jump in and around the topics depending on what is most urgent for you and your child.

You don't need to read the book cover to cover in linear order.

How long should you spend completing each part and the accompanying stages?

This will vary from family to family, but in general terms the main thing is not to rush through the different parties and stages without first trying to bed down some of the suggested changes you may like to make.

In the beginning the program is best tackled slowly but methodically. This means at least taking one, if not two weeks for each stage and maybe up to one to two months for each part of the four-partie program. Some families, who already have embedded some healthy foundations outlined in the program, may not need to make as many changes and thus won't take as long to implement other changes.

The main thing is that you feel like you and your family are learning new ways to live healthier on your Ride to Life and also having some fun doing so. If there are stages you find particularly difficult then don't rush though them and ignore the fact that you have reached a barrier. This is a sign that you need to think more carefully and diligently about why this stage presents such a challenge and openly discuss this with your family to try to find a solution. If after concerted effort the barrier seems impenetrable, then consider going around it and trying another direction as long as you feel it is moving you forward in other aspects of your new journey to better health.

Follow the Just One Thing rule

I devised the **Just One Thing** rule, as a guideline, to help people avoid becoming overwhelmed as they commence and continue on their recovery.

The **Just One Thing** rule means you focus on learning and integrating one new behaviour or habit at a time, rather than trying to learn multiple new things simultaneously. By approaching things this way, you have the best chance of integrating a new behaviour or habit. I've learnt people are less likely to stick with a new action if they have too much going on. Apply this approach to the new behaviours and skills you learn in the book. And remember: if nothing changes, nothing changes.

As part of the Ride to Life Program the **Just One Thing** rule also aligns with the concept of a One Percent philosophy. This suggests that big changes are harder, but shorter, smaller changes made more often and consistently are easier. For example, micro 'one percent changes' all add up over time to big changes that are often more sustainable. Micro changes can add up to mean macro results.

Do the KINIMS!

Another feature of the book is the liberal use of KINIMS.

What's a KINIM? Something I created to help you!

A KINIM is my very own self-styled word that integrates two other words: maxim and kinetic.

- A 'maxim' is a principle used to make a decision.
- The word 'kinetic' means keeping in motion and having positive energy.

A KINIM is about the principle of making a decision and then once decided using the momentum of forward motion to keep going with that decision.

A KINIM then is a piece of advice or an exercise to help you focus on a health change that can help your family keep moving on your healthier life journey. I have shared these KINIMS with my clinical patients for many years and found they work extremely well as reminders to keep us on track.

To make the most of your investment of time and effort, I recommend a couple of things. Firstly, do the exercises described in the KINIMS. It might sound obvious, but it would be easy to gloss over them, thinking you don't need to do them or you'll come back to them later.

The second thing I recommend about the exercises, and all aspects of the program outlined in the book, is to approach everything with complete honesty. This might sound simple, and it is, but it's not easy. Complete honesty about our behaviours is tough and requires courage. For some it may be the hardest work they've ever had to do. Remember that for a healthier, happier life for you and your family, your complete honesty, and that of those around you, is necessary.

The third and final thing I recommend is you make a commitment to yourself and your child. Again, simple, but not easy. Commitment confers responsibility upon us. Personal responsibility is an essential ingredient on the road to recovery. When we're on a bike, it's up to us whether we stay mobile. We must keep peddling or we will fall over. It's the same with commitments. Promises are frequently made but easily broken, especially when something easier or better comes along. Simple does not always mean easy. It's tempting to think we can deal with it later or it doesn't really matter right now. I'm here to remind you addressing the causes of obesity in your child does matter. Their life depends on it. In many ways, your life does too.

Download and sign your Parental and Family Commitment pledge to start, continue and finish your Ride to Life and join the Ride to Life Program for better health and life 'wealth' for your family and connection to your community.

Check the icons

Throughout the book you will find important, useful exercises, references and resources. These are identified by icons. Use these as a guide to taking action and developing your own knowledge and wisdom.

This icon denotes the resources which are available on the Ride to Life website: childhoodobesityprevention.com.au. Available to everyone who purchases a copy of the book, these resources are important tools for helping you stay on track. Make use of them.

Throughout the book, there are video resources you can refer to that explain certain exercises. You can access the videos on the Ride to Life website: childhoodobesityprevention.com.au.

The **Just One Thing** icon is a reference to focusing on just one thing at a time. As I've explained earlier, it's to remind us that as we're learning and integrating new behaviours, and we need to focus on just one thing before moving onto the next thing.

 The KINIM icon highlights the exercises in the book. These exercises are an essential part of creating new behaviours. Make sure you do them!

I encourage you to keep these things in mind as we hop on our bikes and start this journey, beginning as we do with an understanding of where we are right now. Start to think where you would like your family to be after each day, week, month and year on this healthier journey you're embarking on and keep your commitment to them and to yourself.

Ride to Life Commitment

The _____ Family Health Challenge

I/We _____

the parent(s) or guardian(s) of _____

_____

do solemnly commit to undertaking the necessary changes, small and large, that are required for breaking my/our child and family's Cycle of Obesity.

    I understand that this commitment I/we make to start, continue and complete the Ride to Life Program for the better health and well-being of my/our child and my/our family. I recognise that this is the most important thing I/we can do in our lives as a parent/guardian.

_____	_____	_____
parent/guardian 1	*parent/guardian 2*	*child 1*
_____	_____	_____
child 2	*child 3*	*child 4*

Date: _____ / _____ / _____

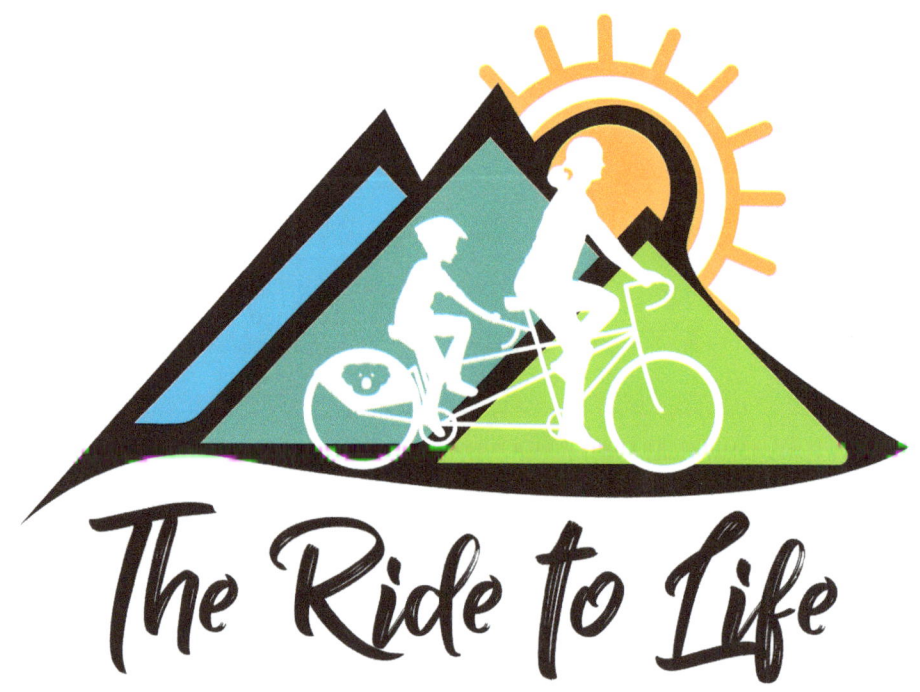

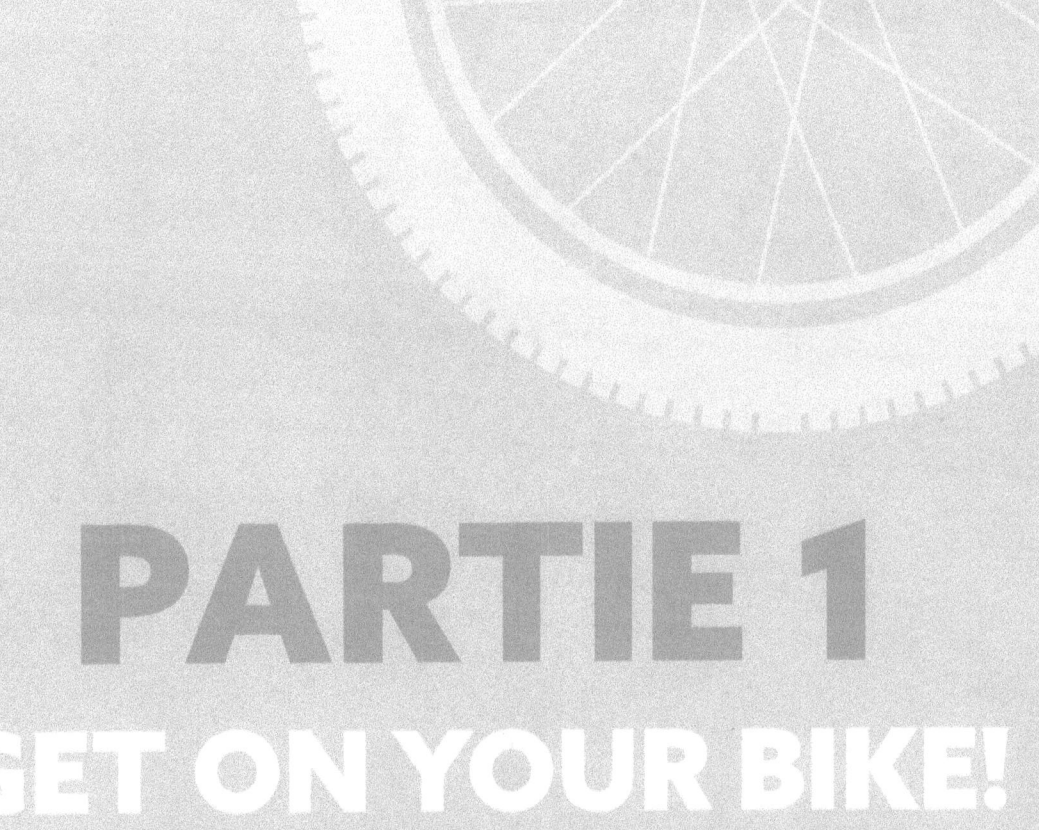

PARTIE 1

GET ON YOUR BIKE!

Taking responsibility for where you are now

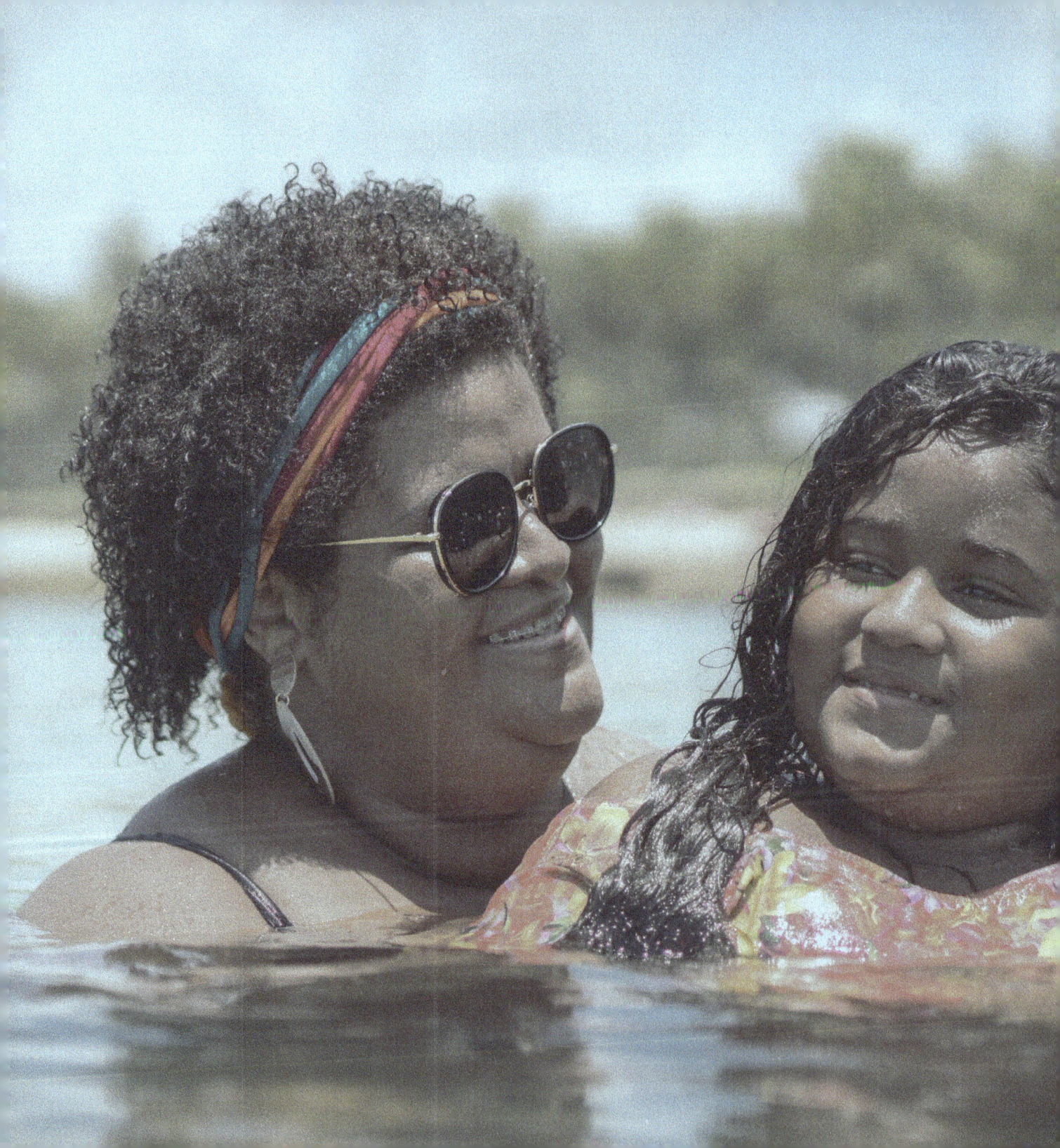

Stage 1

Get honest:
understanding where you are and why

> *Honesty is the first chapter of the book of wisdom.*
>
> Thomas Jefferson (1743-1826) – Third President of the United States of America

No journey can commence without a clear understanding of the start point. Before we do anything then, it's vital we understand where you and your family are right now. Getting honest is critical if you, your child and family want to reclaim better, healthier lives.

In Stage 1, you will:

- Learn the importance of getting honest about the reality of your child's situation.
- Review your family's state of health, taking an integrated approach and reflecting on the various aspects that contribute to the overall picture.

Where are you?

If I were to see you in my clinic, the first thing I would ask you to reflect on is where you and your family are right now. Even before I asked about hopes for treatment, understanding the current situation is a vital first step. To help with this exercise, I have developed a simple questionnaire that uses a one-to-five scale. Among other things, the questionnaire asks questions about:

- Your family's current level of stress
- General fitness i.e. how physically active you are as a family

- Food practices, including shopping, cooking and eating
- Daily and weekly routines, taking into consideration the demands of family life
- Sleep habits, understanding that quality rest has important healing power
- Social supports, looking at who you turn to for emotional and practical support.

The Getting Honest Questionnaire

This first part is for parents and caregivers. There is another section for children later in this chapter.

The Getting Honest Questionnaire requires that you score a response to the following questions from one to five. Do this by circling your response. As you answer the questions, enter the number that corresponds to your answer in the tally table below. Once you've answered all the questions, tally the scores and that number will be a measure of your family's health and wellbeing. The questionnaire score is just an indicator about priority areas you might turn your attention as you move towards a healthier life for your family.

Home

Q1 How would you rate your family's current level of stress? (i.e. reflecting you feeling a sense of control of your family's life)

1	2	3	4	5
High		Medium		Low

Q2 Does your family cook, share and enjoy most meals together around the dining table each week?

1	2	3	4	5
Rarely/never		Occasionally		Most days

Q3 As a family, how often do you have takeaway, frozen and junk food each week?

1	2	3	4	5
Most days		Occasionally		Never

Q4 How physically active are you together as a family each week and weekend?
Do you go to park for ball games, walks, ride your bikes together, swim in summer etc.?

1	2	3	4	5
Rarely/never		Occasionally		Most days, inc. weekends

Q5 How supportive do you feel your family is in addressing your family's health challenges?

1	2	3	4	5
Not at all supportive		Supportive sometimes		Supportive

Q6 How often do you buy fresh living food, like fruit and vegetables for your family?

1	2	3	4	5
Rarely/never		Some weeks		Every week

Q7 How often do you use a weekly routine to organise your family life?

1	2	3	4	5
Rarely/never		Some weeks		Every week

Q8 Do your children (if old enough, for example five years or older) have set chores to help around the house that they need to do complete each day/week? Are there any consequences for the children if they do not complete their assigned chores?

1	2	3	4	5
No		Yes, but there are no consequences		Yes, with consequences

Q9 Do you and your partner share the housework and childcare responsibilities?

1	2	3	4	5
No, one person does the majority or all housework and child-care responsibilities		Somewhat		Yes, we equally share all housework and childcare responsibilities

Q10 Do you and/or your partner/spouse regularly raise your voice/use physical force to get attention or make a point in the family?

1	2	3	4	5
All the time		Occasionally		Never

Q11 How often do you set behavioural boundaries for your children and stick to them?

1	2	3	4	5
Rarely/never		Sometimes		All the time

Self: mind, body and spirit

Q12 As parents, what is your own level of health and physical and mental fitness?

1	2	3	4	5
Not healthy or fit		Moderately healthy and fit		Healthy and fit

Q13 How often do you and your partner/spouse spend time together away from the children?

1	2	3	4	5
Never		Occasionally		Often at least every week

Q14 As individuals and within the family, over a week do you get adequate rest and sleep?

1	2	3	4	5
Rarely/never		Some weeks		Every week

Q15 How often do you engage in a one-to-one conversation with your child/children where you're not providing an instruction or discipline?

1	2	3	4	5
Rarely/never		Sometimes		All the time

Community

Q16 How often does your family attend a community group, church or external organisation (e.g. sports club, music group, Scouts or Girl Guides) to pursue hobbies or interests or community events?

1	2	3	4	5
Rarely/never		Some weeks		Every week

Q17 Do you personally or your spouse/partner participate in, or volunteer, as a coach or leader in any school, sporting, religious, charity, or community group?

1	2	3	4	5
Rarely/never		Some weeks		Every week

Work

Q18 Do you feel a pressure to work long hours, leaving you little time at home with the family?

1	2	3	4	5
Every week		Some weeks		Rarely/never

Q19 How often do financial concerns impact the way your family can live healthily?

1	2	3	4	5
All the time		Occasionally		Never

Q20 How often do you say 'Yes' to someone when you really want to say 'No'?

1	2	3	4	5
All the time		Occasionally		Never

Enter your scores in the table below and calculate the total number.

Question	1	2	3	4	5	6	7	8	9	10	11	12	13	14	15	16	17	18	19	20
Score																				
TOTAL out of 100																				

How did you go with the questionnaire? Review your total score and assess where it sits relative to the following:

- Scores between 75 and 90 indicate you are on the right track, while >90 suggest that you are probably not being totally honest with yourself – but maybe you are!
- Scores between 50 and 70 indicate you have some good things in place, but there's more work to do.
- Scores less than 50 mean that it's time to prepare for a healthier Ride to Life!

Remember, it doesn't matter so much what your score is; it matters more that you have an honest appraisal of where you and your family are now. The score gives you an indication of areas where you may be able to focus initially to bring about change, e.g. being more active as family, eating real fresh food rather than processed, packaged foods and being more connected to your local community and to your children through better communication and use of time.

Having this information clear in your mind at the start of the journey will make all the difference to the outcomes. Importantly, you'll be able to measure how far you've come. You'll also have a clearer picture of what you're working towards. For now, it's enough that you have taken the first step on your journey.

The Life Cycle Questions for Children

Now for child-specific questions, which highlight challenges in your child and their relationship with the rest of the family. Most children seven years or older should be able to honestly answer these questions with some guidance.

CQ1 Do you have set chores or jobs your parents expect you do every day in order to earn pocket money or as a regular part of helping around the house to contribute to running the home?

1	2	3	4	5
No		Yes, but only once or twice a week		Yes, every day I am expected to do my chores

CQ2 What sort of snack would you most commonly have if you were hungry in between main meals?

1	2	3	4	5
Sweet biscuits or packet of chips or other packet snack most days		Sweet biscuits and chips, but only once a week		Raw veggies like carrots, cucumber, fruit, or sometimes an egg

CQ3 During dinner time do you wait till everyone is finished their meal before leaving the table?

1	2	3	4	5
No		Yes, but only sometimes		Yes, all the time

CQ4 Do you have takeaway food often?

1	2	3	4	5
Yes, we go to McDonald's and KFC every week, so have takeaway food at least two to three times a week		Yes, but only once a week		My parents do not allow me or my family any takeaway food

CQ5 Do you eat a piece of fruit and vegetables such as carrots, cucumbers, broccoli and salad every day?

1	2	3	4	5
No, I do not like fruit or vegetables at all		I usually have one piece of fruit and some vegetables at dinnertime		Yes, I love eating fruit and have four to five different vegetables a day

CQ6   What drink do you have every day ?

1	2	3	4	5
Juice or soft drink		Sometime juice but mostly fresh water		I only drink water or fresh unflavoured milk

CQ7   What is your favourite thing to do after school and on the weekends?

1	2	3	4	5
I like to watch TV, play video games or watch YouTube on my iPad or computer		I like to read and draw and only am allowed to watch less than two hours of TV or iPad time a day		I love to be active outside and play my sports a few times during the week and on weekends

CQ8   What time do you get to bed and sleep on school nights ?

1	2	3	4	5
I am up after 10pm, sometimes later, most school nights		I usually get to bed by 9pm most school nights		I am expected to be in bed by 8pm most school nights so I get at least 10 hours of sleep a night

CQ9   How do you get to and from school each day ? Do you walk, scooter or ride your bike, or take the bus and/or train, or get driven to school?

1	2	3	4	5
I get driven to and from school by my parents		I walk to the bus or train stop to go on public transport to and from school		I walk or ride my bike to and from school

CQ10   When you eat your favourite food at dinner time are you a very slow or very fast eater? Slow means takes at least 30 mins to finish your main meal and very fast means less than 10 mins.

1	2	3	4	5
I finish my main meals in 5–10 mins		I usually take about 15–20 mins to finish my main meals		I take my time and usually finish my main meal in about 25–30 mins

CQ11 When you eat your dinner do you sit in front of the TV or computer while eating or around the dinner table with all your family?

1	2	3	4	5
I love watching TV when I eat my dinner		I usually sit at the dinner table with my family but the TV is still on as it has my favourite show		I eat at the table with my family with no TV on

CQ12 Do you belong to any clubs – sporting or otherwise – that you go to every week to play and meet friends?

1	2	3	4	5
No, I do not belong to any clubs		I attend the school clubs and also sometimes go to PCYC or Scouts to do fun things		Yes, my family and I belong to sports clubs, and/or a church group and also other fun community clubs like PCYC, YMCA and Scouts

Enter your scores in the table below and calculate the total number.

Question	1	2	3	4	5	6	7	8	9	10	11	12
Score												
TOTAL out of 60												

How did you go with the questionnaire? Review your total score and assess where it sits relative to the following:

- Scores between 40 and 60 indicate you are on the right track!
- Scores between 20 and 40 indicate you have some good things in place, but there's more work to do.
- Scores less than 20 mean that it's time to prepare for a healthier ride to life!

Body Mass Indicator (BMI)

A BMI is a measurement of body size and is one way to assess whether a person's weight falls in a healthy range.

A BMI is a screening tool that can indicate whether a person is underweight or if they have a healthy weight, excess weight, or obesity. It is calculated using height in metres and weight in kilos.

Keep in mind that a BMI is just a number. You must take it into context along with the information revealed from the questionnaire. What's important is your overall picture of health.

Input your child's details into the online calculator at: pro.healthykids.nsw.gov.au/calculator/. This excellent calculator gives you a good idea of the weight status of your child, and if overweight to what degree. It might be an eye opener for some parents! It also allows calculation of the BMI of the parent's to indicate their weight status.

If you do not have access to the internet the BMI charts are shown on the following page.

The kids' site also provides growth charts to help you get a sense of where your child sits for their height and weight in comparison to their peers.

Record the BMIs of the whole family in the table below.

Name	BMI	Assessment (underweight, overweight, obese)

Completing this assessment may have been distressing. I have found this assessment often leads to a lightbulb moment where the parent is shocked into seeing how severely obese their child is. I find it also results in a deeper understanding about how serious the consequences are for their child. While it might be difficult to absorb now, the importance of this information to bring about change cannot be underestimated.

Some children I see in my clinics are what I call my '10 X kids'. This means their age in years multiplied by 10 equals their current weight in kg!

For example, a 10-year-old child weighing 100kg or a five-year-old weighing 50kg.

Boys BMI chart from age 2–18 years[6]

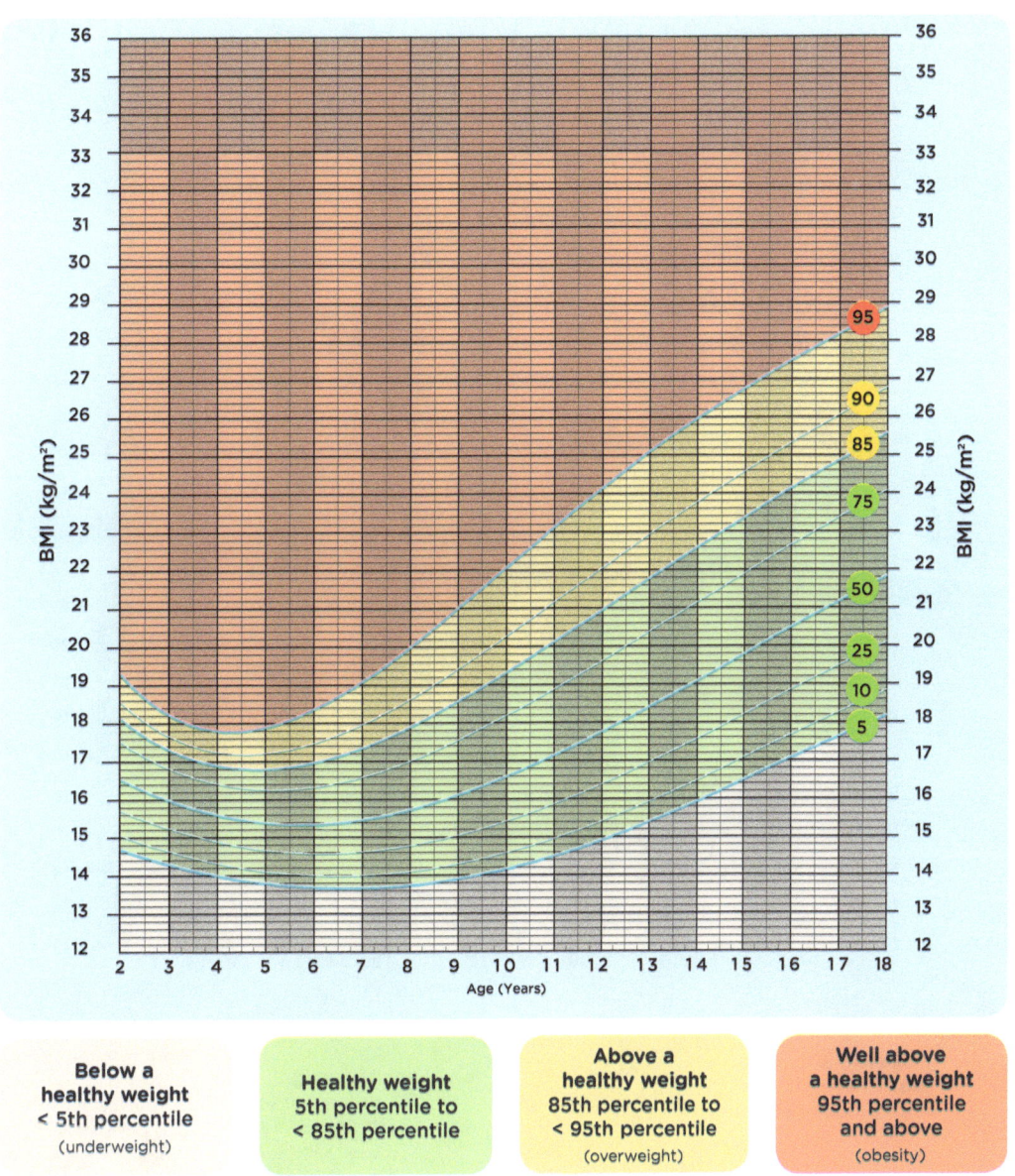

Sourced from Healthy Kids for Professionals at pro.healthykids.nsw.gov.au/resources/. Reproduced by permission, NSW Health © 2020. Original BMI charts from Centers for Disease Control and Prevention (CDC) (2000).

Girls BMI chart from age 2–18 years[7]

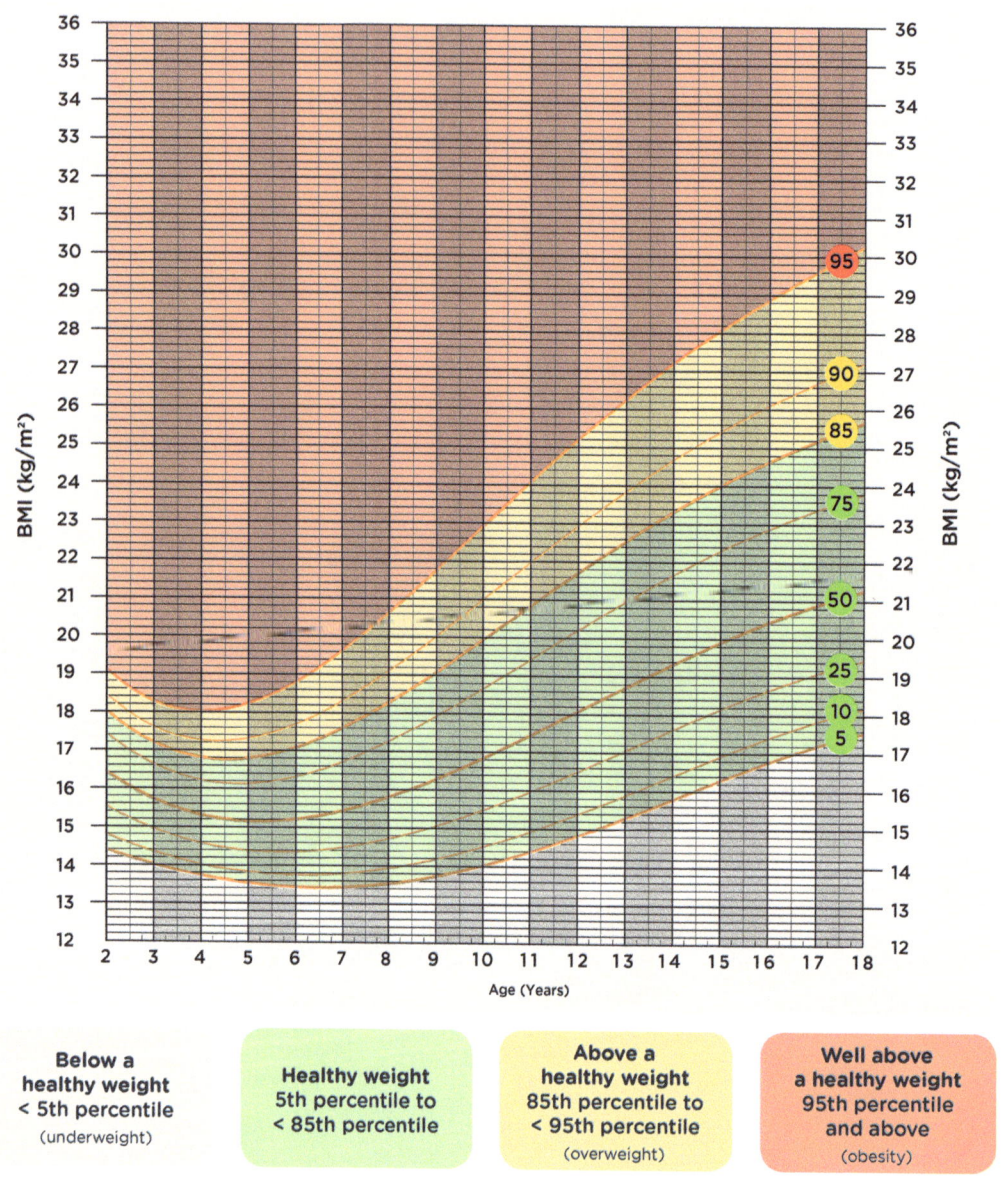

Sourced from Healthy Kids for Professionals at pro.healthykids.nsw.gov.au/resources/. Reproduced by permission, NSW Health © 2020. Original BMI charts from Centers for Disease Control and Prevention (CDC) (2000)

These children are in serious medical trouble, and I see such kids routinely in my clinic. They and their parents do need help and compassion.

Those children with less severe obesity, but nevertheless still in the obese range (if older than five years of age) I call my 'Five X kids', so a ten year old weighing 50kg or five year old at 25kg.

You can look at the weight growth charts from the CDC to get a picture.

Boys

www.cdc.gov/growthcharts/data/set1/chart03.pdf

Girls

www.cdc.gov/growthcharts/data/set1/chart04.pdf

A frequent question parents and their referring doctors ask me about their child is could there be a genetic or hormonal cause for their severe obesity.

The simple answer is yes definitely, as I do occasionally see children present with hypothyroidism or rarely other genetic syndromes that influence body size which sometimes are associated with other health problems such as developmental delay, kidney or neurological problems.

However the excessive weight gain of the overwhelming majority of the children and their families that I see in my clinic is due to their high intake of ultraprocessed packaged 'fake' toxic food and sedentary behaviour with lack of daily regular physical activity. Then add on top of this the ill-effects on a family of chronic psycho-social stress on positive parenting, sleep, mental health and social and family connection, you can see why it is not easy for some families with obesity to make healthy changes for themselves.

Resources

Make sure you also get across to the Ride to Life website and access all the online resources that are available there.

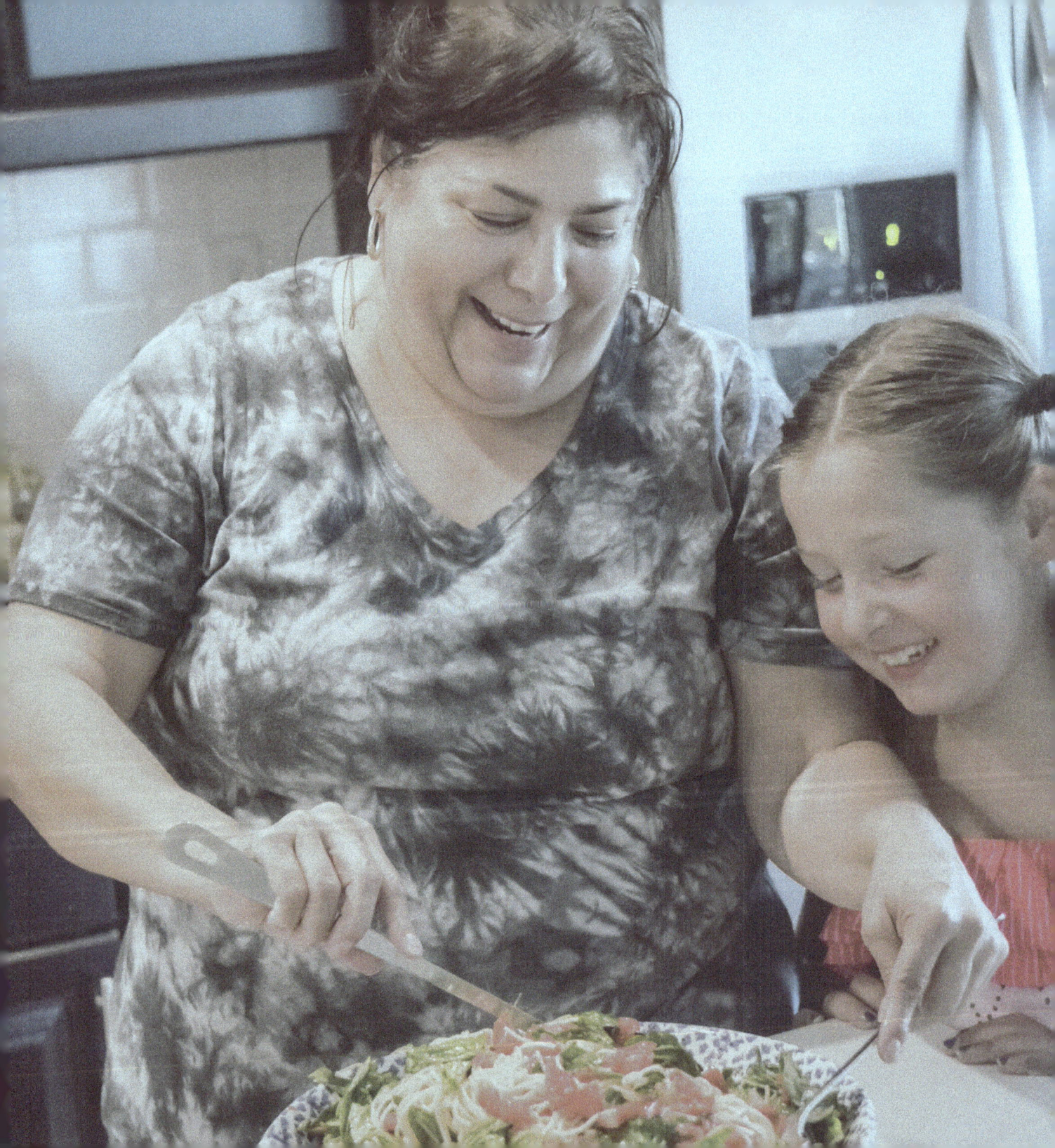

Stage 2

Decision time: committing to a healthier life

I have always struggled to achieve excellence. One thing that cycling has taught me is that if you can achieve something without a struggle it's not going to be satisfying.

Greg LeMond, American professional road cyclist and triple winner of
Le Tour de France in 1986, 1989 and 1990. The USA's only winner of Le Tour de France.

At this point, its imperative you're clear about the **'Why'** for your journey, or as Dr Koala likes to call it the **'Big W'**. Without knowing your **'Why'**, you'll never be able to hold firm to your commitment. Your resolve will dissolve at the slightest hurdle. A very personal thing, the **'Why'** for bringing about lasting change is different for everyone. For some people, it will be fear of diabetes. For others, it may be concerns about heart disease. Some parents want to avoid their child experiencing the same emotional trauma related to their own weight journey during childhood or adolescence. Almost all parents in this situation are fearful about their child's long-term health and future wellbeing.

In this stage, you will:

- Get clear about your decision to commit to healthy changes.
- Understand the growth mindset needed to undertake this commitment.
- Understand the reality of any challenging journey.

Why commit?

When I'm preparing for a big ride, I take time to clarify in my own mind why I'm doing the ride. If I didn't, I can tell you that I'd most certainly give up when the going got tough. And believe me when you're riding up a mountain with a 10 percent gradient or more, you do question why you're making yourself suffer!

On your journey, it will be the same for you. When the going gets tough – like when your child and/or other family members complain about food changes, or when family members criticise you – it can just feel easier to give in and give up. Without your '**Why**' very firmly fixed in your mind, you will be tempted to give in. When this happens, there is the secondary fallout of living with the disappointment that you've 'come off your bike'. The other side of the equation is you've also lost momentum and direction. Restarting is hard, and in many cases, people don't. They give up for good. Don't be that person. Get clear about your '**Why**'. Your child's life depends on it.

Getting honest about your fears

What is your biggest concern about not addressing your child's health issues?

Is it a fear your child will die before you? Is it a fear that your child is continuing your family's cycle of obesity and its associated health effects such as diabetes, cancer and heart disease?

Take time to reflect deeply on what your biggest fear is. You may find this causes you to feel emotional. If it does, great. This is actually good, as it means it has hit a nerve and it's therefore significant for you and a more compelling reason for change.

Use the space below to write out your biggest fear.

What are your biggest hopes and dreams for your child?

Reflect upon what kind of future you hope your child can have if you can break the cycle of obesity. Focus on their physical health, happiness and wellbeing and how they might achieve their own special potential.

Drafting your 'Why'

As you draft your '**Why**', frame it in positive language that gives you and your family hope. For example, you could write:

*My '**Why**' for committing to a healthier life is to ensure that my child has the best chance of reaching their full potential and living a healthy, happy, enriched life.*

Avoid using any negative words in your '**Why**'. For example:

*My '**Why**' for committing to a healthier life is I don't want my child to get diabetes.*

That may be true, however it will be more effective for you (and your child) if the language is written positively.

Get other family members involved

If you have a partner, have your partner do this too if possible and then share your concerns and '**Whys**' with each other. This is an important exercise for staying on track, as it establishes a vital bridge to understanding where each of your family members is coming from.

Consider if your child is mature enough to complete this exercise. If they are, say, ten years or above, have them do this too. From this age, a child starts to develop a sense of independence and can think through some of their feelings about their life. It's also an important tool for encouraging age-appropriate responsibility.

Make a note here of your most significant hopes for the future if you can commit to a healthier life, and fears for your child if their obesity is not addressed. Once you've done that, write down your '**Why**' for making a commitment to a healthier life.

My most significant hope for my child is:

My most significant fear for my child is:

My '**Why**' for breaking the cycle of obesity and committing to a healthier life is:

Sign and date:

Visit the Ride to Life website to download copies of this that you can print out and also share with other members of your family.

Get creative

Take your '**Why**' and put it somewhere you can see it and read it every day.

I find that a vision board is a wonderful way of communicating a big goal or dream we have for ourselves. For you, it's an opportunity to get creative. You can do it with the resources you have around the house. Get some blank sheets of paper, old magazines, colouring pencils, paints and crayons. Imagine what you would love life to look like for you and your child. (For example happy at home and school with lots of smiles! Being part of a school music band or sports team or acting class.)

Be sure to include your '**Why**' on the vision board. Perhaps put it in the car, on your mirror in the bathroom, or on the fridge. Let it become your mantra. When you're walking along, repeat it. If you're waiting in line, think of it.

Hold on to your '**Why**' as it will sustain you through the inevitable challenges that will arise. It will also strengthen your resolve when you've achieved a win.

What if you're riding solo?

If you're unable to engage other members of the family to commit with you, don't let discouragement lead you to abandon the journey. Instead, seek support outside of the family. Recognise too that it can be difficult to be a prophet in your own home. Often our own family is the source of greatest resistance, including our partner, parents, siblings and children. While it's ideal to have support from your family, the reality is it doesn't always happen. To bring about change, you need to be committed enough to go ahead anyway, with or without them.

There's no doubt a lack of family support can be demoralising, but it doesn't mean you go without support; it just means getting help elsewhere. Your support people don't need to be professionals. They can be someone you trust enough to lean on and know they'll listen when you need it. You may also choose to obtain professional support for yourself; however, a trusted, supportive friend may be all you need, or have access to, right now. It might take a little time to discern who that person is, but keep looking until you find them, remembering you may need more than one.

> I provide more information about choosing your support team in stage 8, so you may want to refer to that before you share your '**Why**' with another person.

Change starts with you

Here's what I know. When a parent (hopefully both parents) makes a decision and a commitment to caring for themselves, there is a direct correlation between that commitment and an improvement in their child's health. There is also less resistance to change. As hard as it may be to accept, if you focus on your own health and wellbeing first, this will directly impact your child's health and your family's health.

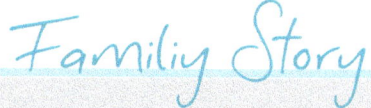

Familiy Story

Mother Power

Karolina is a beautiful three-year-old girl of Samoan background.

Her grandfather was very sick with end-stage diabetes and heart disease (and eventually passed away six months after I first saw Karolina in my clinic). This had an amazing, motivating effect on Karolina's mother to make changes at home to improve Karolina's health and excessive weight.

At age three years she was 26kg, well above the normal healthy range, in the severe obese range with a BMI of 27kg/m² (see page 34 for growth chart to illustrate severity of obesity).

Karolina was the youngest of four children and her parents were divorced. There was family history of obesity, type 2 diabetes and heart disease on her mother's side and type 2 diabetes on the father's side.

Karolina's excessive early childhood weight gain was due to high intake of packaged, processed foods and takeaway foods. With substitution of these fake foods for real fresh home-cooked foods, raw vegetable snacks, less sugary breakfast cereals, more water and more physical activity in play group, over six months Karolina's mother was able to make sustainable family changes. This was despite being a busy single mother with a family of four children, some of whom being older were not happy to have their junk food – chips, chocolates and sweets – removed from the pantry and fridge! The changes led Karolina's weight to remain stable over six months, so when I saw her last she had lost a small amount of weight from 25.7kg to 25.4kg and with excellent height growth her BMI fell from a peak of 27kg/m² to 22.9kg/m². Though this weight and BMI is still well above the 99th percentile, the resolve of Karolina's mother has been strengthened by the tragedy of her own father's death from diabetes and wanting her children to avoid this common pathway of ill-health that has been part of her family's life stories. She decided it was not going to be her or her beautiful daughter's story from now on!

Bringing about that change, and seeing the difference in her daughter, compelled her to keep going and stick with her commitment to breaking the cycle of obesity in her family.

Keeping your commitment

If I use the analogy of an endurance bike ride, like Le Tour de France, the team of riders know the route they are going take each day. They also know the final destination. The goal is to reach Paris and ride on the Champs-Élysées and around the Arc de Triomphe. What the competitors don't know is what will happen, minute by minute, each day. The riders will face potholes, crashes, crazy fans, punctures, fatigue, mechanical failures, and physical and mental challenges.

It will be the same for you on your Ride to Life.

Hold the picture of your important '**Why**' in your mind, but know there will be many challenges, some totally unexpected. But remember, as you continue, you will also receive unexpected support and rewards along the way that bring you great joy and hope too. These things will sustain you and often appear in surprising ways.

Take one day at a time

A commitment to a healthier life is just that: for life. But if you look too far ahead, it can be easy to feel overwhelmed. I remind people in my clinic that it's taken many years for them to reach the point of crisis and it may take several years to unravel it. That said, I can reassure you I've seen many families who've embraced a healthier life and consequently seen wonderful changes in their child's health within a much shorter timeframe.

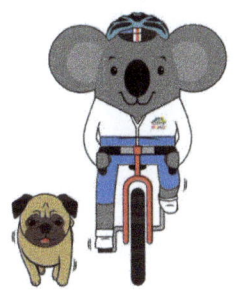

For Le Tour de Koala!

While it's a cliché, it's for this reason I encourage you to keep your '**Why**' in mind, but take one day or one week at a time. In doing so, you make life more manageable.

In our Ride to Life Program, you'll find 100 ideas for implementing the **Just One Thing** rule. Just one small thing at a time is much easier than making big changes and yet small steps can lead to big results.

Having healthy rewards

It takes courage to make decisions that lead to change. It also takes courage to stick with them. Now you've decided to start a journey towards a healthier life, take a moment to acknowledge the significance of your decision. It really does have the potential to transform the lives of you and your family. Though this may seem to be a small step, each milestone is worth celebrating. Such celebrations are essential along the way. On Le Tour de France, this occurs at the end of every stage of the three-week race, when the race leader receives the *maillot jaune*, or yellow jersey, that is worn proudly on the next stage. Think of the healthy reward as your own yellow jersey that gives you extra strength and power for the next stage of the Ride to Life.

Make a list of healthy rewards for yourself. Have this on standby for those moments when it's time to celebrate. Knowing your healthy non-food rewards will help keep you and your family on track. If you have trouble thinking of some healthy rewards refer to Dr Susan Albers' book *50 Ways to Soothe Yourself Without Food*.

Here are some suggestions to get you going:

- Buy yourself a bunch of flowers
- Listen to your favourite music and dance to it
- Get a massage
- Plan your next family holiday
- Watch your favourite comedy and have a good laugh
- Take the kids for a day at the beach or park for a walk or ride.

Make a list of your healthy rewards here. Over time, you can continue adding to it as you find kinder and more loving ways to reward yourself for your progress.

My list of healthy rewards includes:

1.
2.
3.
4.
5.

Be sure to add these to your vision board where you can see them.

See also the section on self-care in stage 8.

Resources

Print out your '**Why**' and place it somewhere visible, together with your list of healthy rewards.

Notes

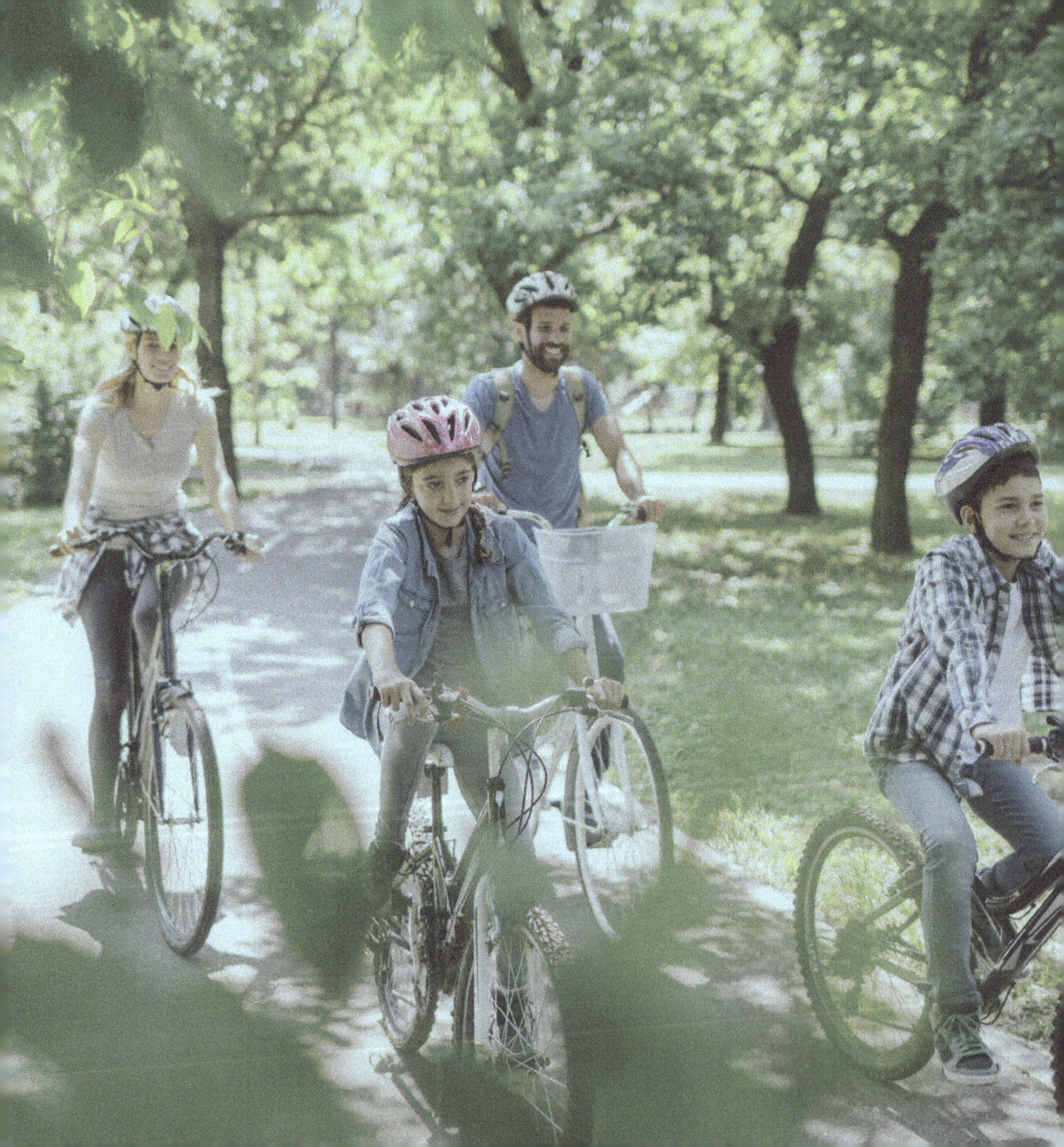

Stage 3

Getting ready for change: preparing for the ride to a connected life

> *Change is not something that we should fear. Rather, it is something that we should welcome. For without change, nothing in this world would ever grow or blossom, and no one in this world would ever move forward to become the person they're meant to be.*
>
> Sri B.K.S Iyengar, Yogi and Founder of Iyengar School of Yoga

You've no doubt heard the saying that if nothing changes, nothing changes. Change is hard and no one really likes it but in this stage we will explore the different ways to make change possible.

Part of the process of claiming a connected life is as an opportunity to change any habitual thinking that's not serving you any longer. Why is it important to let go of this old thinking? Well, your old thinking is what got you here. Your new thinking is what will position, and keep you, on the road to recovery and hopefully a healthier and happier connected life.

In this stage, you will:

- Learn the importance of prioritising the work required to break the cycle of obesity.
- Understand why it's necessary to make changes in routines – yours and your family's.
- Understand challenges arise when we make changes, but learn these challenges can be managed when we have the right tools in place.

Make change your new friend

If you're anything like the other almost eight billion people on the planet, there's a good chance you'll have an aversion to change. As humans, we love the familiar. I get that. There's no denying change can be difficult. This is especially so in the early stages of breaking the cycle of obesity, but as we discard old behaviours and replace them with more constructive and positive ones, change becomes easier to manage. As you become more fluent in the new behaviours, they become second nature. Ultimately, you end up with a more enjoyable way to live.

Now that you have made the commitment to a healthier life, it's important that you prioritise and allow time and space for change to happen. Many of us feel overwhelmed in our daily lives and like we are constantly running from A to B. Being 'time-poor' is a common challenge for parents and families which makes taking on changes difficult. Part of the change process requires you look at your and your family's current routines and how you can create some time and space to implement changes to improve the health of your family. These changes in routine don't have to be permanent. The important thing is to actually make some space so you can focus on your health. As with other activities in the book, I recommend reflecting on this task with honesty – I call it the big 'H'. H can stand for many positive things and it can become your power chant to success!

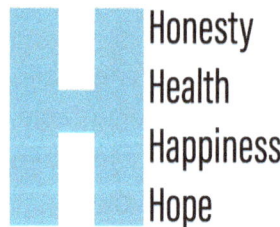

H for honesty; for health; for happiness; for hope!
The big 'H' – remember this!

Look deeply into the areas of your family's routines, or possibly lack of routine, to determine where time and space can be created to first allow you the chance to implement some small positive changes.

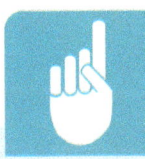

A word of caution about change

The journey you're embarking upon is the most important of your life. For changes to be sustainable and have maximum impact, it's vital you pace yourself. Apply the **Just One Thing** rule. Not only does this make it more manageable for you, it is also a wonderful example for your child to follow. It gives them permission to pace themselves as well, rather than feel pressured and stressed by the process and an unhealthy need to 'do everything' at once.

As part of the Ride to Life Program we have identified that there are a number of ways you can start to make small changes in your life as a family and as individuals. Including things relative to personal care and time out, whether you're the parent, grandparent, or additional support person in your family, the need to make small changes and know that these can each lead to bigger outcomes is vital. Big changes are often unsustainable because they require buy-in from everyone. But if everyone focuses on committing to the **Just One Thing** rule within your family, there will be a gradual growth in the mindsets of all towards change for better.

This is also about doing what you each can as individuals as well as collectively within your family.

Review the family's routine

What does your normal day and week look like? Include the weekend in your considerations. A great deal can be understood about what we prioritise by looking at how we spend our time – and that is the purpose of this exercise.

How is the family's time spent? What are the essential things that need to be done each week that cannot be changed? While this may appear to be set, do keep an open mind about how your daily routine is currently arranged and prioritised. If you and your family do want to start a healthier journey, a key part of whether you will be successful in making sustainable change is being courageous and open to doing things differently than you have been!

This will require negotiation between you and your partner and the children, but as the parent, YOU need to make the final decision, not the child or adolescent, though positive constructive input is welcome!

I don't underestimate that for many families this is the hardest thing to do. To negotiate the need for healthy changes in your family, when perhaps your adolescent children and maybe your partner or the grandparents are dead against your efforts and deliberately sabotage you.

This is why it is so important that you as the parent and primary agent of change need to foremost ensure your own mental and physical health is prioritised before you start this new challenging journey. Without this fundamental foundation the 'straw house' will definitely fall down and with it the three little pigs inside when that first ill wind comes along from the Big Bad Wolf!

As the old saying goes: 'When the plane is going down, make sure you put your own oxygen mask on first before you start helping others with their needs!'

As a simple example, I always explore with the family how the children get to school and home again. Most children these days are driven by their parents to school, often on the way to work for one or other parent. If old enough and with help, could the child learn how to take public transport, saving the parent valuable time, but also teaching the child or adolescent valuable lessons about taking responsibility, being independent and being organised? There might be a flow-on effect of the child wanting to get to bed earlier to have a good sleep which might promote a healthier breakfast that is not rushed. You might encourage them to walk to the bus stop, whereby increasing their incidental physical activity. They might have the chance to talk with friends who might also be on the bus, increasing their social time.

I even suggest to families to explore the possibility of driving to school but stopping a kilometre away from the school and having the child walk the rest of the way with mum or dad, which gives the parents valuable time to talk and walk with their child, and some few thousand extra steps in their day!

Use the format on the next page to identify how time is used by each family member. Look for where time is wasted or where there is an imbalance of time on a particular activity.

	PARENT			CHILD		
	Before work 6–9am	Lunch hour	After work 5–9pm	Before school 6–9am	After school 3–6pm	Evening 6–9pm
Monday						
Tuesday						
Wednesday						
Thursday						
Friday						

	PARENT			CHILD		
	Morning	Afternoon	Evening	Morning	Afternoon	Evening
Saturday						
Sunday						

For example, if one child plays soccer six days each week and another child is unable to get to other activities and is suffering as a consequence, now is the time to explore how each individual's needs can be integrated into the household schedule in a more balanced way. It doesn't necessarily mean stopping the first child from playing soccer six days per week, but it may prompt you to consider alternative ways of achieving the same outcome. It might mean asking a friend or relative for help with transport once or twice a week to allow you to attend to the physical needs of your other child or children.

So, let's get started.

Looking at all areas of your family's routine, can you identify time that could be more effectively used or saved?

How much time? Make a note of this below. For example, could you start a carpool to a school commitment with another child's parent? Could you change the time of a commitment to make it more convenient for the whole family? Even half an hour can ease stress levels. If piano lessons aren't really convenient on a Tuesday night, could they be changed to Saturday morning? Could you consider taking a term off from an activity while you focus on your health?

Looking at the division of household tasks, is there a fair and equitable division of domestic duties? Could the balance be readdressed to allow more time for some members of the family to focus on other health-related issues? Are the older children, especially the adolescents, being given responsibilities and duties around the house to teach them independence and value of teamwork?

Many parents today have become like hotel managers doing everything for their children and these children grow up with fewer life skills and an attitude of expectation without effort! Doing chores properly gives both children and their parents a sense of achievement and pride in their work. It also teaches a child about responsibility and provides a sense they need to contribute to the running of their home.

I could save time by:

1.

2.

3.

I could ask for help with:

1.

2.

3..

The benefits of doing making these changes are:

1.

2.

3.

School holidays and a special mention of the summer Christmas holidays

The end of the year and start of the year are often especially challenging for some families with obesity, as some holiday periods can be two months or longer. Also, there are numerous important national, cultural and religious celebrations when families get together where food is abundant, rich in sugar and perhaps not as healthy. In addition, though Australians love the summer beach time, many do not have easy access to summer water sports. However, being out of the normal school and physically active routines, especially if the parents are not on holidays, older children and adolescents are commonly home alone being very sedentary on their TV and computer screens with altered unhealthy sleep patterns and over-snacking.

I routinely see children in my clinic who come back in February having gained three to four kilos over the summer holidays since their last visit, undoing all the good they have done up till the end of the year.

Family Story

Holidays don't mean taking a holiday from being healthy and active

Calvin is an 11-year-old Chinese boy. His mother brought him to see me because of his excessive weight gain, being 64.2kg at nine years and eight months with a body mass index of $30.8 kg/m^2$ in the severe range. He was the only child. He lived with his mother, who was healthy weight, and his grandmother. His mother has pre-diabetes and is taking metformin to prevent the development of diabetes. This was the mother's '**Why**', her motivation to help her son get to a healthier weight. Calvin already had signs of abnormal blood liver function with tests suggesting fatty liver disease, which is now the commonest cause of liver transplant in young people.

His father lives overseas in China where he works and returns to Australia to be with his son and wife a few times a year. Calvin regularly visits his father and grandparents in China on school holidays. This is where he is indulged with lots of takeaway food or restaurant eating and inevitably gains weight of three–four kilos over the summer holidays in China. As in many cultures, in China being overweight is commonly considered a sign of good health and this is typical of many older Chinese persons' cultural beliefs.

Calvin's weight gain during early childhood was related to high intake of processed and takeaway foods, juice intake, relative lack of physical activity and excessive screen time, more than two or three hours a day on iPad, watching TV and playing games on Playstation.

> Neither parent was overweight but had a history, like many Asians, of pre-diabetes.
>
> Calvin was encouraged to be more physically active and reduce screen time, and eat slower and more mindfully (20-minute rule for main meals) with smaller portions. The parents were asked to be more aware about the effects of excessive holiday eating in China and to plan for this and engage his relatives to not overindulge him with sweets and takeaway food. Despite their best intentions, the family found it difficult to deal with the needs of these healthy boundaries for their son.
>
> He was encouraged to only drink water and eat more real, fresh rainbow food, especially vegetables and one or two pieces of fruits per day, while reducing his intake of processed packaged foods and unhealthy snacks (e.g. biscuits, chips, sugary cereals, white bread).

Avoiding this Christmas–summer holiday effect requires forward planning and thinking of the scenario in an objective way to ensure the kids remain active and eat healthy portions of real, fresh food and not be overindulged by their extended family. But *how*, you might ask. First you have to get serious about avoiding situations where your family overindulges beyond the most important family occasions at Christmas and New Year celebrations! Eating like this is not going to be a winner! Many schools, organisations and sporting clubs run summer holiday activity programs. Of course finances must allow for these extra activities, but ensuring your child does not fall into the summer-time trap is crucial for maintaining your Ride to Life.

Commuting and travelling

In this step, make notes about the time and method taken to travel to and from school and work for each individual. Include work and school commitments.

DAY	AM TRAVEL			PM TRAVEL		
Monday						
Tuesday						
Wednesday						
Thursday						
Friday						
Saturday						
Sunday						

Use this as an opportunity to identify areas of imbalance or conflict that prevent either parent from undertaking healthier behaviours (and thereby taking the lead). For example, if your work commute requires you travel an hour each way, it reduces the available time for self-care and connecting with other family members. Over a working year, if you worked from home one day a week, this could equate to roughly 100 hours that could be spent focusing on your health and breaking the cycle of obesity in your family. Undoubtedly, that would be time well invested.

Work

Another area that warrants closer scrutiny is work.

Obviously, we all need money to live. Within families today, it's a juggling act for most parents and carers to manage the financial health of the family. If you are working full-time, is it possible to adjust working arrangements to create the necessary time and space to allow you to focus on implementing changes? Remember, adjustments don't have to be forever. They may only be required for the time it takes for positive changes to occur. What kind of flexibility you can consider will depend upon your vocation and the nature of your industry. Consider a variety of flexible arrangements that could give you more time at home during the hours the family is at home.

Consider:
- Hours of work (changes to start or finish times)
- Patterns of work (split shifts or job sharing)
- Locations of work (working from home)

Here are a few examples:
- A nine-day fortnight
- Working from home one day a week
- Leaving work early once a week and picking the kids up to go to park for a fun active session before dinner
- Changing your hours to 8am to 4pm, or even 7am to 3pm and being home when the kids get home from school to talk, help them with homework or go for a walk or bike ride
- Taking a later shift to ensure that breakfast and school drop-off go smoothly
- Taking on light duties
- Accessing long-service leave
- Accessing carer's leave
- One full day off every month

Long hours

Many parents battle against the expectation (from their boss and themselves) that they must work beyond the hours of 9am to 5pm. Depending on the nature of your job and your industry, long hours may be standard. In order to keep your commitment to your health and your child's health, you may need to find a way to negotiate around the need to work long hours with your boss (see below for more on this) but also with yourself. You are battling a serious health crisis. Your child's life depends on you keeping your commitment to good health, and you need time and space to do that. Ask yourself if you really need to work as many hours *right now*. There are certain projects and deadlines that are important and need extra attention, but if long hours are habitual for you, every day, every week, every year, you will need to find a way to change that while you focus on changing your and your child's health. For some people, committing to coming home on time every night may be the most they can give on the work front, and that's OK. The important thing is to find a way to maximise your time at home with your family.

Talking to the boss

I recognise that reducing or altering hours of work can be a real challenge for some parents for a variety of reasons. Whether you're parenting as a couple or solo, it can also be a challenge to negotiate with your boss, particularly if they're not understanding of your personal circumstances. Having these life-changing conversations requires preparation and consideration. This means preparing your case in advance, pre-empting responses, and being ready for objections. When people in my clinic face this challenge, I recommend they present their position as a win-win for both parties.

What kind of flexibility could be available to you? Remember that you are battling a health crisis. Depending on your relationship with your boss, sharing the details of the situation may help garner their sympathy and understanding. There is no shame in what you are doing. Quite the opposite. You are asking for the time and flexibility to care for a family health crisis. If your child was seriously unwell with a more recognisable illness, your work would be legally obligated to grant you time off to deal with it (carer's leave). You have every right to at least open a conversation on the topic of flexibility while you tackle this health crisis.

> Do you want to be the parent on whose gravestone is etched, 'They were very good at their work'?
>
> Or the parent whose gravestone reads, 'They were a great, loving, present parent'?
>
> I know which words I want on my memorial!

My small story

I reached a crisis point in 2012. I realised work was not fulfilling me as I was missing my family and not caring for myself physically or spiritually. I was working as an academic at the University of Queensland as well as putting in hours at the busy clinical practice at the Mater Children's Hospital in Brisbane. However my family was based in Sydney, which required that I commute between Sydney and Brisbane every week.

Unsustainable and unhealthy, I decided it couldn't continue, but I only started to make change after I fractured my hip when I fell from my bicycle. The six weeks of forced time-out allowed me to reflect on my values and life priorities, particularly as they related to my family, work and self-care. After giving things considerable thought, I approached my respective bosses at the university and hospital.

I explained my situation and proposed that I begin working fewer hours, thereby allowing me to spend an extra day in Sydney with my family and have time for self-care. The difference this made to my mental, emotional, physical AND vocational wellbeing was immeasurable. Life became more manageable, and that is what we are looking for here through this reflection exercise.

If your work is unwilling to grant you any flexibility even for a short time, you may consider changing jobs for another with hours and conditions that are more conducive to implementing sustainable changes. Though this fallback option is probably not one you may at first prefer, sometimes we have to do things that seem unpleasant and difficult, but with every door that closes, another door of opportunity always opens – you just have to have your eyes and heart open and be ready for that door of opportunity to open! At least that is my philosophy for a happy life!

While each person's circumstances are different, I encourage you to give this area the time it deserves. There may not be an immediate solution, and that's OK; however, I feel as we open up to the possibility that a certain pathway is right for you and your child, the way for you to negotiate more time away from work will come to you. I encourage you to stay open to the possibilities, as this always allows unexpected doors to open, even when others close.

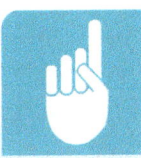

Tips for tough conversations

The secret to tough conversations is being prepared. Here are some tips for negotiating arrangements that will help you fulfil your commitment to a healthier life.
- Prepare your case, outlining the benefits to all involved in the new arrangement. The benefits might include financial savings, but they might also demonstrate improved productivity, better morale, and so on. Be sure to consider the benefits to others, that way you can show you're not just thinking about yourself.
- Ask to trial the new arrangement for a short time, with the potential for extension to be considered at the end of the trial. That way, both you and your boss can assess whether it's working or not. It also gives both parties an opportunity to re-negotiate if it isn't.
- Look at having at least one 'Plan B'. What are your options if the new arrangement doesn't work out? Knowing you have a fallback position will give you confidence. You might start with trying to negotiate for a day off a week, but you might be happy to concede to a nine-day fortnight or to just work from home once a week. You might simply arrive at an understanding with your boss that you may need to leave early more often than normal.

Stay-at-home parents

The pressure and busyness for those at home can be just as challenging as for those working full-time. A stay-at-home parent *is* often fighting numerous fires and racing against time to get a thousand myriad things accomplished every day, many of which are invisible to the other family members. It's not uncommon for a stay-at-home parent to put themselves last on the priority list. A stay-at-home parent is often perceived as having 'plenty' of time to pick up extra family tasks as they're 'at home all day'. The care of elderly family members, for example, is often automatically delegated to stay-at-home parents, even when other members of the extended family are capable of completing such a task.

If you are at home part-time or full-time, as part of this exercise consider ways in which you too can create time to prioritise your health. Remember: the work of a stay-at-home parent *is* work. Think of it this way: any task that you would have to pay someone else to perform if you didn't do it *is work*. Watching TV isn't work but taking family members to the doctor is. To create time for you to focus on your health may mean calling upon other family members to attend to tasks that they normally wouldn't be asked to or at least creating more balance as to who is responsible for what. Could there be a rotation for who hosts family dinners? If housework and childcare isn't equally divided between the parents, now may be the time to reassess this. (I realise that this can be a can of worms in itself!) If finances allow, consider hiring a cleaner to do a fortnightly or monthly clean or a babysitter for a few hours on the weekend. Making time may also mean letting some tasks fall by the wayside.

Later we will talk about the importance of saying 'No' to allow you to say 'Yes' to the things you truly value (see stage 9). This applies equally to office-working and home-working parents. Also see the section on self-care in stage 8.

Remember that children can and need to be encouraged to take on responsibilities by doing chores that contribute to the running of your home. Simple things like dishes, laundry, kitchen tasks are great ways for them to help out and start to learn long-term domestic skills. After all, they will be running their own adult lives one day. Kitchen tasks such as helping with dinner preparation is also a time saving for you and helps them to be involved in learning good food and table habits.

School

'Over scheduling' has become more common among kids today. School hours are frequently extended beyond 9am to 3pm by after-school commitments like sports training, music lessons, tutoring and, of course, lots of homework. Considering the commitments your child currently has, and without eliminating something that gives them real joy, is there some way to create more time and space for them to focus on their health? Could they take a term or semester off from something? This may allow more outdoor playtime with the siblings or with you, Mum and Dad! Yes, what a joy that would be!

Food preparation and food-sharing habits

In this step we will identify the main person responsible for shopping and cooking for the family. To do this, answer the following questions.

Who is the person responsible for the family food shopping? ☐ Mum only ☐ Dad only ☐ Mum primarily but Dad sometimes
What habits do you have around shopping for the family? For example, do you shop at the same time/place each week or is your shopping more ad hoc?

Do you make a shopping list? If you do, is it your habit to stick to it? ☐ Yes ☐ No	Do you have a meal plan that informs your shopping list? ☐ Yes ☐ No

Do you work to a food budget?
Does your family eat takeaway? How often and how much money do you spend on it? What percentage of your total food spend is allocated to junk food?

How much time do you spend doing the family food shopping (including travelling to and from the shop)?	Where do you shop? At a fresh-fruit grocer or a major supermarket chain?
How much time do you spend preparing your meals?	Who helps with meal preparation?

How many main meals do you spend eating together?

Breakfast on weekdays ☐ out of 5 and on weekends ☐ out of 2

Lunch on weekends ☐ out of 2

Dinner on weeknights ☐ out of 5 and on weekends ☐ out of 2

Planning

Here's the golden rule to work by when it comes to food shopping and breaking the cycle of obesity: failing to plan is planning to fail.

If you're not planning your shopping trips, including what you'll buy and when you'll shop, you place yourself at increased risk of over-shopping and filling your basket with processed, packaged and high-sugar foods and drinks which contribute to the continuation of the cycle of obesity.

I often see people in my clinic who initially resist the change to putting more structure around this aspect of their family's lives. However, once they've tried it for themselves usually, after a very short time, they see beneficial effects from their efforts: a reduced grocery bill, healthier meals, and more enjoyable family time. The reward then drives their ongoing commitment to sustainable, constructive change. It is the structure and discipline around food and its preparation that makes the difference in families.

Family Story

The Khans KAN!

One of my most rewarding encounters with a family who needed help was with a four-year-old Pakistani boy.

He was the youngest of six children.

They were a beautiful family, but had been living a very unhealthy life, with basically all the children aged from four to 15 years eating junk and takeaway food most nights of the week, with high sugar and saturated-fat intake.

This poor nutrition led the youngest child of the family to be about 28kg in weight and have a BMI in the extreme range equivalent to an adult with a BMI of about $45–50 kg/m^2$. This little boy then developed gall stones and a gall bladder infection or acute cholecystitis secondary to the gall stones. He had to undergo an emergency cholecystectomy which was very traumatic for him and his family.

There was a strong family history of obesity and type 2 diabetes on both sides of the family, and this little boy already had evidence of severe insulin resistance and fatty liver disease – all precursors of type 2 diabetes!

I only saw him once in my clinic but the parents totally embraced our healthy message for the whole family. The mother became the primary agent of healthy change and embraced lifestyle changes and our recommendations in regard to eating healthy nutritious real rainbow food with fruit and vegetables and immediately stopped the junk food, takeaway diet! They also became more physically active as a family.

They shopped only for fresh, real food at their local vegetable market and by stopping buying the junk food and takeaway meals they saved themselves $400 per month! The father lost 15kg in six months!

I did not see the family for another seven months. But, when I did, I did not recognise the little boy; he had changed so much. Firstly, he was smiling, when before he was sad. In fact the whole family were happier, with the older children all supportive of the healthy changes they had made, with each playing positive roles. The little boy basically then started growing into his weight not gaining any further weight such that as he grew taller his BMI fell from an extreme obesity level to a moderate obesity level. Most importantly, his signs of risk for diabetes such as the insulin resistance and fatty liver disease markers on blood tests totally disappeared and normalised. In other words all his metabolic complications were completely reversed while his behaviour around food became normal, eating less and not always being hungry, anxious and moody like he was before when he was eating the toxic junk and takeaway food. The parents were ecstatic about his marked improvement and motivated to continue their healthy journey while saving money as well!

How to change your family's food habits if you want to break the cycle of obesity

In a very practical way, when it comes to changing your family's food and life, we need to start working on one meal at a time. Reaching the point where you're able to do this means completing a Healthy Home Food Scan, whereby you examine the contents of your fridge and pantry. When I explain this to my patients I say to them, if the food is in a packet there's a very good chance it won't be as healthy as something grown or produced naturally in living healthy soil!

In the Healthy Home Food Scan, we look at the fridge and pantry. Applying a simple is best approach, the aim is to declutter these important spaces in your home, thereby allowing you access to the healthiest foods possible, and empowering you to avoid foods that are temptations and/or create unnecessary food fighting.

Even before you rearrange or discard all the unhealthy foods and drinks in your fridge, section off a zone of your fridge that is at eyesight level and easily accessible. I suggest this is the space located at the middle right-hand side of the fridge. Make this zone the place where your first healthy foods go and can be easily spotted and found. Over time, this area will expand and eventually cover the whole fridge and freezer.

Clean out the fridge and pantry

Prepare your family for this important exercise by discussing why it is important to not keep unhealthy fake foods and drinks in the house.

'Out of sight means out of mind.' When you keep these processed foods in the home by hiding them or locking them away in the cupboard, it gives the message to your kids that it is still OK to have them in the house. They'll start to think, 'Well they can't be that bad can they?' Then those little minds will find them either directly or wear you down till you relent in a weak moment!

Open your fridge and pantry and take photos of how they are right now. Look closely at the contents.

Throw out (yes, in a garbage bag) any foods that are unhealthy, keeping only those that will nourish you and your family. Remember, in general, 'healthy' food is fresh and real food that is not in a package or in a can!

The kinds of foods you will throw out include:
- Any sugar-sweetened beverages (e.g. soft drinks, juices and cordials)
- Lollies, biscuits and chocolates, unless it's dark chocolate (which does have some health benefits in small quantities)
- Sauces, such as tomato, barbecue, and sweet chilli sauces
- Condiments, such as mayonnaise
- Pre-packaged snacks, such as muesli bars, fruit straps, fake cheese dips, chips, muffins, donuts
- Low-fat, sugar-sweetened yoghurts and desserts
- High-sugar-content cereals – read the food label and any packaged foods greater than 5g of total sugar per 100g goes in the rubbish
- White-coloured foods, including white bread, white rice, white flour, white sugar and white potatoes
- Artificial sweeteners, which have been shown to increase fat production and the risk of type 2 diabetes

- Canned foods, such as soups, spaghetti, baked beans (which may have bisphenol A or BPA in the lining of the can, which is an endocrine disrupting chemical (EDC) shown to cause hormonal imbalances leading to increased risk of diabetes, obesity and cancer[8]), though some canned vegetables and tuna can be part of a healthy pantry
- Dried foods, such as two-minute noodles (which have a huge amount of trans fat in them derived from palm oil), dried fruit, flavoured chips and snacks.

Once you have removed these items from your fridge and pantry and disposed of them, you should be able to see some space in your home for healthier options, but also space in your heart and mind to breathe and feel a sense of achievement.

Before you panic and think you've nothing to feed your family, I encourage you to read on as we continue to explore your shopping habits, and dig into menu planning and food shopping in more detail. We will go into more detail about healthy food and nutrition in stage 5. For now, we're going to stay focused on the habits and routines that will keep you on track.

Delete your takeaway apps

Apps like Uber Eats, Menulog and Deliveroo make ordering takeaway so simple you don't even have to make a phone call or leave the house. With your credit card on file, it can be easy to order and never even think about how much you're really spending. Check out your latest credit-card statement to see how often you have been ordering takeaway and how much you have been spending. Then delete the apps! If it's not on your phone, then the temptation will be removed. Replace these unhealthy apps with the FoodSwitch app from The George Institute for Global Health in Sydney which gives uses a traffic light system to give you healthy alternatives to much of what you buy in your local supermarket.

Check your shopping receipts

As a secondary aspect to this vital decluttering exercise, there is enormous value in reviewing receipts from your regular grocery shopping. Insights into your family's management habits around food can be gained by collecting these receipts over two weeks (including any restaurants and takeaway food). Using a red-coloured highlighter, identify unnecessary and unhealthy food items in your shopping basket.

By including this activity in the clean-up of your pantry and fridge you are gaining a 360° view of what's really going on. It also means you must honestly face what's really feeding into your family's cycle of obesity.

The process of reviewing your family's food is a bit like decluttering your wardrobe. However, the big difference is that your life, and the life of your family, depends on it. If you stay true to your why, it will empower you to follow through with the job of removing the unhealthy foods. Once you've completed this exercise, you will feel an immense relief in the knowledge that you have drawn a line in the sand from which you can move forward.

In my clinic, patients have the benefit of a supportive dietitian who can help empower the patient's family. If this is not option for you, enlist the help of a support person, who understands your family's situation and your why, and to whom you've given permission to help you hold firm to your resolve of breaking the cycle of obesity.

After emptying your fridge and pantry of the unhealthy food and drink, you can begin to plan what food will replace that which you have discarded. You can do this by working with a menu plan and a shopping list.

What's a menu plan?

A menu plan is a weekly plan for your family's meals. It allows you to plan ahead for breakfast, lunch and dinner, and for snacks.

By taking time to do this work upfront (even before you've set foot in the kitchen), you reduce the likelihood of deviating from your pathway to a healthier, happier life for you and your child. There are many benefits to a menu plan:

- A plan minimises the amount of food you need to buy, thereby reducing waste and expense.
- It reduces the chance you'll take shortcuts when you may be stressed or stretched to the limit, and then find yourself in the queue of the closest fast food drive-through.
- A menu plan will also flag to other members of the family there is a clear structure to meals. Accordingly, it should be respected as such, with all family members participating in this daily ritual.

Recipes

Among the many resources on the Ride to Life website, there are also recipes you can use, so check these out as well. Apply the **Just One Thing** rule and start with one recipe you feel you can manage. Once you've mastered that one, move onto the next. Use the recipes on the website until you feel confident enough to start developing your own.

I have received various recipes from Louise Elliott (www.louiseelliott.com.au and www.KidsGetHealthy.com.au), founder of CommonHealth Kids and the author of the book *The Amazing Army* and the *Amazing Army Kids Nutrition Show*, and also lunchbox ideas and recipes from Bel Smith of www.therootcause.com.au. The aim is to empower children and their parents to make healthy and better food choices, especially at school. Bel has developed The Mad Food Science Program, which she and her husband Israel have rolled out nationally in more and more primary and secondary schools around Australia. I would highly recommend you read Bel's new book *The Lunchbox Effect* to support your family.

Lunchbox menu plans

As you are planning out your week, don't forget to consider what will go in your child's lunchbox. Make sure you have options on hand rather than trying to decide on the day and having to hand over money for the tuckshop.

Do not include sweet or unhealthy items as a 'treat' for your child or as a gesture of love. Nourishing them with real food is a stronger statement of love.

As a parent you are most likely responsible for organising food for school. Keep in mind that you are responsible for supplying the food and your child is responsible for whether or not they eat it. But if your child is old enough, say from pre-school age, they may participate in choosing healthy foods for their lunch as part of them learning to take responsibility for their health.

Here are some examples of healthy lunchbox items:

- Fruit: apple, banana, grapes, strawberries, cherries, pear
- Vegetables: carrot sticks, celery, snow peas (served with hummus or other healthy dip)
- Cheese cubes or sticks
- Falafel balls
- Lentil patties
- Hard-boiled eggs
- Plain or natural yoghurt frozen overnight
- Slice of vegetable frittata
- Cold homemade pizza
- Rye-bread sandwich with lean meat and vegetables (lettuce, tomato, grated carrot)
- Water (no cordial, juice or soft drink)

 For samples of menu plans and items for lunchboxes, please visit the Ride to Life website.

Make a date with yourself

For the first few weeks of implementing your menu plan, you will need to set aside a time where you can focus without interruption or distraction from this important planning task. Because this time is so important, right now I want you to pull out your phone and schedule a date with yourself once a week for the next four weeks to do your menu planning. Then set up a monthly or at least quarterly (change of seasons is a nice time to reflect) time to attend to this activity.

Make this time sacred. It is in this space you will do your important creative and critical thinking about the food that will change and save the life of you and your family. It is worth every ounce of investment you make in it.

Taking this approach might seem like hard work, and, initially, it is. As you develop this new skill, you are applying the same process you'd adopt if you were learning to swim, ride a bike, or speak a new language. It takes time and requires patience. At the beginning, aim to keep your menu plan as simple as possible, while also incorporating enough interest to avoid the inevitable resistance that will come from the rest of the family as new, healthier options are introduced.

This is another activity in which you can enlist the help of your support person. You can also connect with the Ride to Life community. Whatever you do, don't do it alone!

Write a shopping list

Now you've emptied the pantry and fridge of the fake foods and set up a menu plan, it's time to re-stock with the healthier substitutes and ensure you have the ingredients required to produce the recipes in your new weekly menu plan. In stage 5 we will discuss nutrition and define what are healthy foods to feed your family and nourish your child, but for now consider the value of making a shopping list to keep you on track when you buy food. With your new approach to meals and health, you will come to appreciate and value your shopping list. It will be the food 'bible' you'll rely on to plan and prepare life-saving food for your family.

In New South Wales, the Go4Fun free lifestyle program (find them at www.go4fun.com.au) runs healthy shopping supermarket tours, so I strongly encourage you to explore this resource as you commence on the journey to healthier eating.

Food shopping shortcuts

These days many supermarkets offer 'click and collect' or even home delivery at a time convenient for you. By ordering online at your own pace, you'll save the rush and stress of going to the supermarket as well as the temptation to add unhealthy items to your cart.

Bringing it all together to start the change

Now it's time to look at the initial changes you can make to change unhealthy food habits and create new healthy ones that break the cycle of obesity in your family. Here are just a few simple suggestions for commencing the process of change.

1. **Make a shopping list every week.** More than just a list for remembering what you need, a shopping list will assist you with purchase decisions. My philosophy here is: if it's not on the list and it's not a need, don't buy it. But keep it simple, keep it real and keep it economical.

   Making a shopping list requires time and planning. Sticking with the list requires resolve. Make the shopping list your friend and embrace it as a tool to stay on track. Frame the shopping around the guidelines for healthy eating, which emphasise a balance of fresh fruit and vegetables, wholegrains, lean meats and protein, healthy fats, including dairy products.[9] You can refer to stage 5 for more information about how to do this.

2. **Make a menu plan every week.** It will keep you and your family on track for what you're eating and when.

3. **Agree to non-negotiables.** If one parent is responsible for doing the shopping, he or she must stick to the list. Remember, the same rules apply to all family members. Avoid using the weekly food shop as an excuse or way to demonstrate 'love' for your family by placing unhealthy, discretionary foods like chips, biscuits and lollies in the trolley. Highly destructive, this behaviour undermines the good work being done to break the obesity cycle, making it

harder to stay focused on the 'Why' for reclaiming your life. It's also not in keeping with your new philosophy of maintaining a healthy food zone at home.

4. **Eliminate takeaway food from your family's weekly food routine and replace it with life-giving home-cooked meals.** For example, instead of frozen or takeaway pizza, make a pizza at home. Be sure to have the ingredients on hand to do this (i.e. add them to the shopping list) and take time to plan your family's meals ahead.

Try this change experiment

To begin the process for change, identify between one and three actions you can commit to as a start. The priority in most families struggling with the cycle of obesity is around food habits:
- overeating,
- eating processed food,
- buying takeaway food,
- eating large portion sizes,
- eating too quickly and mindlessly.

Consider if one of these food habits affects your family and use this exercise to experiment on how you can effect change.

Apply the **Just One Thing** rule and try one of the ideas listed above (in the list of one to four things for bringing it all together) that you feel will deliver the best outcome for your family. Do it for a month, then reflect and reassess the effect this experiment has had on your family's life.

Consider if it's been positive. If it has, then embed it into your family's routine. Then if you feel confident, start a second experiment and follow the same process. If you don't feel confident going ahead with the change, ask yourself why the experiment didn't work as you'd hoped and design another experiment around the same thing that may have greater success. Check in with your support person and see if they have any suggestions.

Remember to avoid taking too many steps too quickly

Change is best done progressively, by taking small steps, allowing the integration of new behaviour and habits that are setting you and your family up for a healthier, happier life. It will take time. Be patient with yourself and with your family. Expect setbacks. You may start changes but then hit hurdles like, for example, criticism from grandparents who feel you should not stop them giving their grandchildren unhealthy sweets every time they see them. Or a crisis in the family such as a death of a loved one or even a pet! Unexpected upheavals could push you or your child off course. Or maybe simply the school holidays – when healthy lunchboxes and active routines are thrown out the window – may present difficulty. Or you may be challenged when on a family holiday away, especially on a cruise, when takeaway or buffet overeating consumes your family and before you know it everyone has gained several kilograms in weight and guilt! You may also face resistance from other family members who think you are crazy to make these healthy changes, but don't get off your bike.

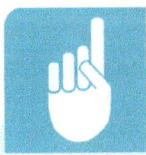

A few words about changing habits

Changing established habits is very difficult, but not impossible.

The secret, if there is one, to changing from an unhealthy to a healthy habit is becoming aware. Through expanded awareness, you can recognise the power of the hook that draws you into the negative habit and the reward that nourishes you to maintain the positive habit. What I mean by the 'hook' is the trigger that leads to a negative behavioural response in you. It could be a comment, situation or person that prompts you subconsciously to respond a certain way.

For example, when faced with a hungry child in a supermarket, your immediate response might be to abandon your healthy shopping list and appease the child's behaviour by putting unhealthy snack foods in your trolley. You do this to avoid the meltdown from the child, save yourself the embarrassment of the public tantrum and avoid judgement from other shoppers. Another hook that many people have is around meal times. In a similar vein, a child demanding more food after having already eaten their evening meal might trigger you to respond inappropriately. You may raise your voice, tell your child off and a benign situation spirals into a heated argument.

New behaviours will feel uncomfortable when you first start them, but they won't feel uncomfortable forever.

Just keep pedaling.

What are your hooks?

What are the hooks that take you off track? Being aware of these hooks means you can put in place measures to prevent you from being 'hooked'. If this is the first time you've thought about triggers or hooks this way, it's a good idea to start by identifying a typical situation that causes you to weaken your resolve around food.

Can you identify one or two major hooks that trigger a negative response in you and could prevent you from staying on track?

Hook	How it stops me from staying on track with healthier behaviours
1:	
2:	
3:	

Avoiding the takeaway triggers

It's one of the easiest things to do when you get to the end of the day, you're all tired, and the cupboards feel bare as you think about dinner while still getting home. The way to avoid the takeaway trigger that is often part of life when those busy days build up is to not only pre-plan your grocery list and shopping, but perhaps take time to pre-prepare extra meals and freeze them for those days.

It's relatively easy to prepare an extra plate of nutritious stew, casserole, or even use your crock pot as a special event on the weekend to ensure your freezer has some additional meals stacked away that only need defrosting and reheating when needed. If you have something like a crock pot, you and your child can also explore which vegetables and meats with a variety of flavours you like. It's a good way to introduce cooking skills to children and an easy way to ensure vegetables get eaten too.

Protein balls are another handy thing to make ahead of time and keep in the cupboard or fridge for those extra snacks that taste good but are filled with nutritional foods. And they are easy to make and modify, experiment with flavours and tastes.

By identifying the hooks that set off undesirable behaviours from you, your child and family, you can plan and practice an alternative set of more positive responses or behaviours that keep you on your healthy journey. For example, you could:

- Delay your response to any request for food by taking three breaths, saying you'll give it some thought, or ignoring the request altogether.
- Respond firmly to any demands or abuse from your child and then move away from them.
- Set up clear parameters around food that is allowed and holding firm to those guidelines.

Rewards

Earlier I referred to the idea of reward and I want to clarify what I mean by this. I don't just mean a thing or treat as a reward. My concept of reward is broader. When I talk about reward in this way, I'm referring to the good feeling or outcome you experience as a result of a newly integrated healthy habit.

For example, you might see improved behaviour from your child as a result of eating more balanced, healthier meals. Consequently, you experience less stress, less food fighting occurs, and you have more time to enjoy each other's company and connect as a family. When this happens, what's really going on is you're starting to reclaim your life. You're starting to break the cycle of obesity. It is as important to know the rewards as it is to know the hooks. By rewarding yourself in healthy ways, you're taking an affirming step towards reclaiming your life.

What reward would you love to experience as a result of implementing your new healthy habit/s? For example, would you like to feel calmer and enjoy a more balanced state of wellbeing? *(Write your thoughts below.)*

The consequences of not establishing these habits is that your family continues to go around in circles, rather than get moving on towards a healthier life. The harsh reality is the cycle of obesity won't be broken and there is less chance of you being able to reclaim your lives.

It's time to get serious

It's not just me saying this. When I see people in my clinic, one of their most significant and common concerns is that *nothing will change and their children will continue their family's destructive cycle of obesity*.

I can assure you that it is only by taking small steps consistently towards your goal of a healthier, happier life that the cycle will be broken. There are no silver bullets, and even if there were, it is much harder to maintain the gains made through rapid-step changes.

It's vitally important you do the exercises in this stage because they will establish the foundations for the change we're talking about. Without strong foundations, it will be difficult to continue building positive, healthy and sustainable behaviours into your family's life. Avoid jumping ahead, thinking you don't need to do this work.

It is critical to your success.

Resources

Make sure you also get across to the Ride to Life website and access all the online resources that are available there. You will find useful tools like a template shopping list, family timetable and other helpful resources designed to help you stay on your Ride to Life.

In his book *Total Leadership*, Stew Friedman talks about the importance of integrating different aspects of life – work, family, health, community – to truly experience a healthy, more fulfilling, connected life. We touch on these concepts here in this stage. You can read further about this in Stew Friedman's new inspiring book that expands his Total Leadership program to helping parents called *Parents Who Lead*.

Checkout this goal tracker template: www.etsy.com/au/listing/260997606/goal-tracker-goal-planner-resolutions

You can also check out the references at the back of the book, where you'll find the links to useful websites, such as www.health.gov.au/health-topics/obesity-and-overweight. There is a huge volume of information about physical activity and nutrition making it well worth the visit. The bonus? It's all freely available to anyone wanting to make changes.

Eat This Much: I recently discovered this great meal planning app (www.eatthismuch.com) through a dietitian friend. If used with nutritional advice from your dietitian or doctor, it will really focus you and your family on how much and what you and your family need to eat to be healthier and lighter! Though designed in the U.S.A I think it is a very educational and practical tool to help your family plan meals based on custom-designed diets and options for adolescents and adults wanting to eat healthier, smaller portions to lose excess weight. Always consult with your dietitian and doctor though if you do use such online resources. Alternatively, download for free this meal plan and shopping list: www.etsy.com/au/listing/162443651/family-meal-planner-kit-printables

Kids Get Healthy: www.kidsgethealthy.com.au founded by nutritionist, author and health entertainer, Louise Elliott. Louise is the creator of the wonderfully fun and educational 'Amazing Army Food Show' for 4–8 year olds.

The Root Cause: www.therootcause.com.au developed by Bel and Israel Smith, an amazing couple and parents themselves, who are transforming the lives of thousands of children and families across Australia through their Mad Food Science program and healthy school lunch box system.

Jamie's Ministry of Food – Learn Your Fruit and Veg program: jamiesministryoffood.com.au/our-purpose/jamie-olivers-learn-your-fruit-and-veg supported by The Good Foundation (jamiesministryoffood.com.au/the-good-foundation)

Stephanie Alexander's kitchen garden program: www.kitchengardenfoundation.org.au

Simply Recipes – a great USA-based healthy fun recipe site: www.simplyrecipes.com/recipes/type/quick

Diet Doctor – for low carbohydrate recipes and advice: www.dietdoctor.com

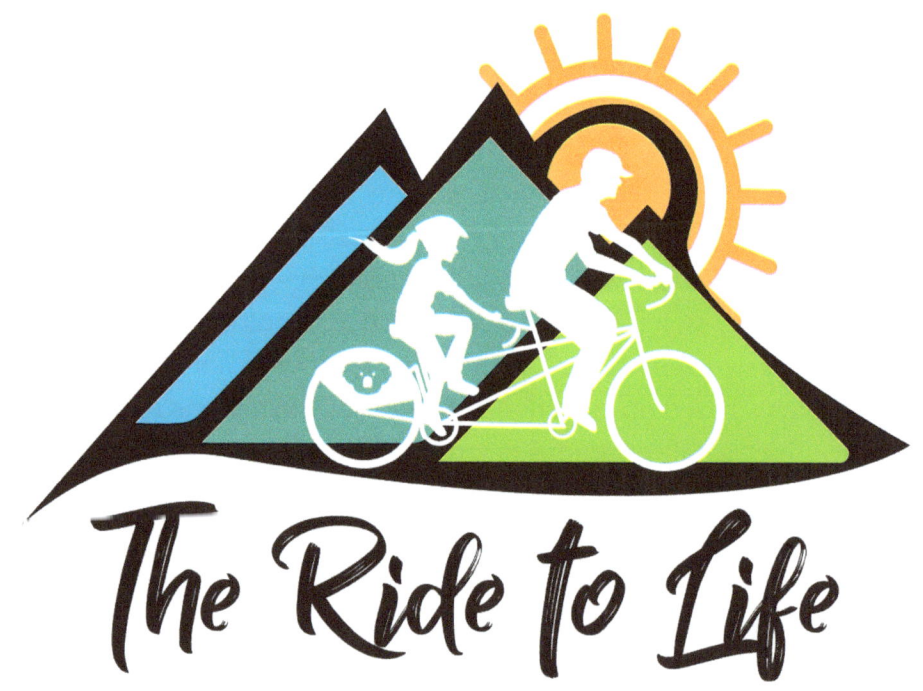

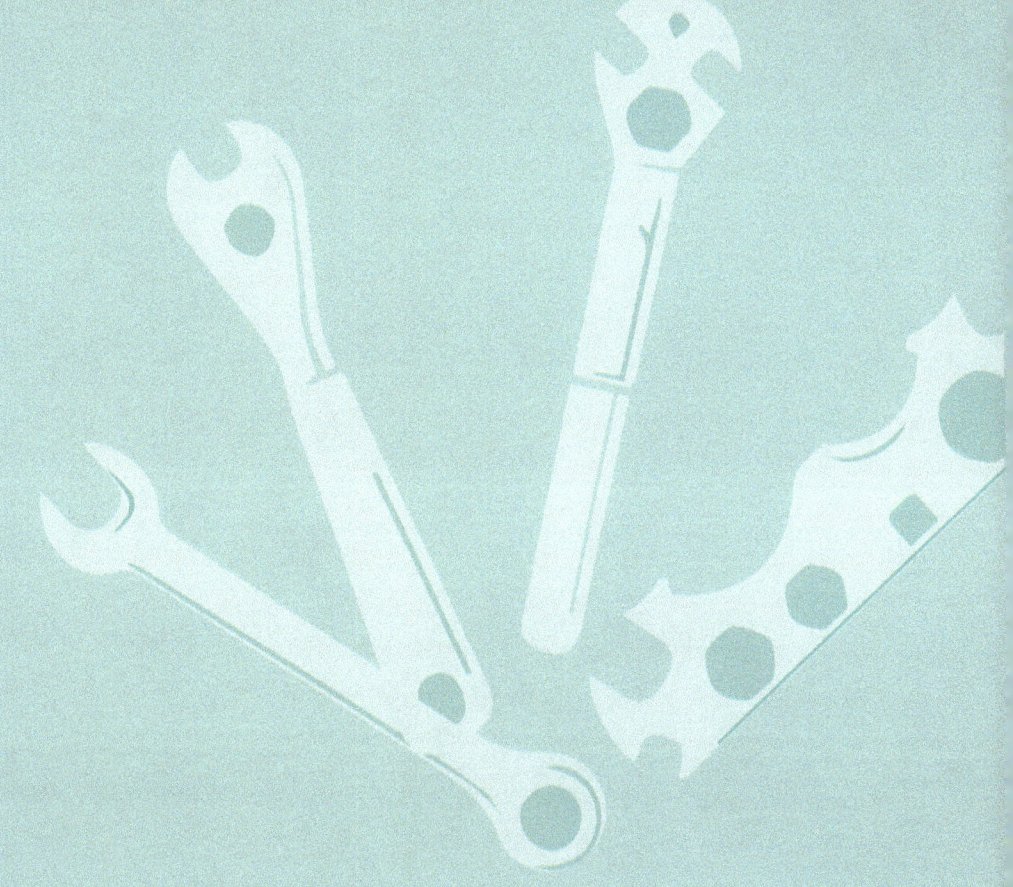

PARTIE 2
IN TRAINING
What it takes to break the obesity cycle for your family

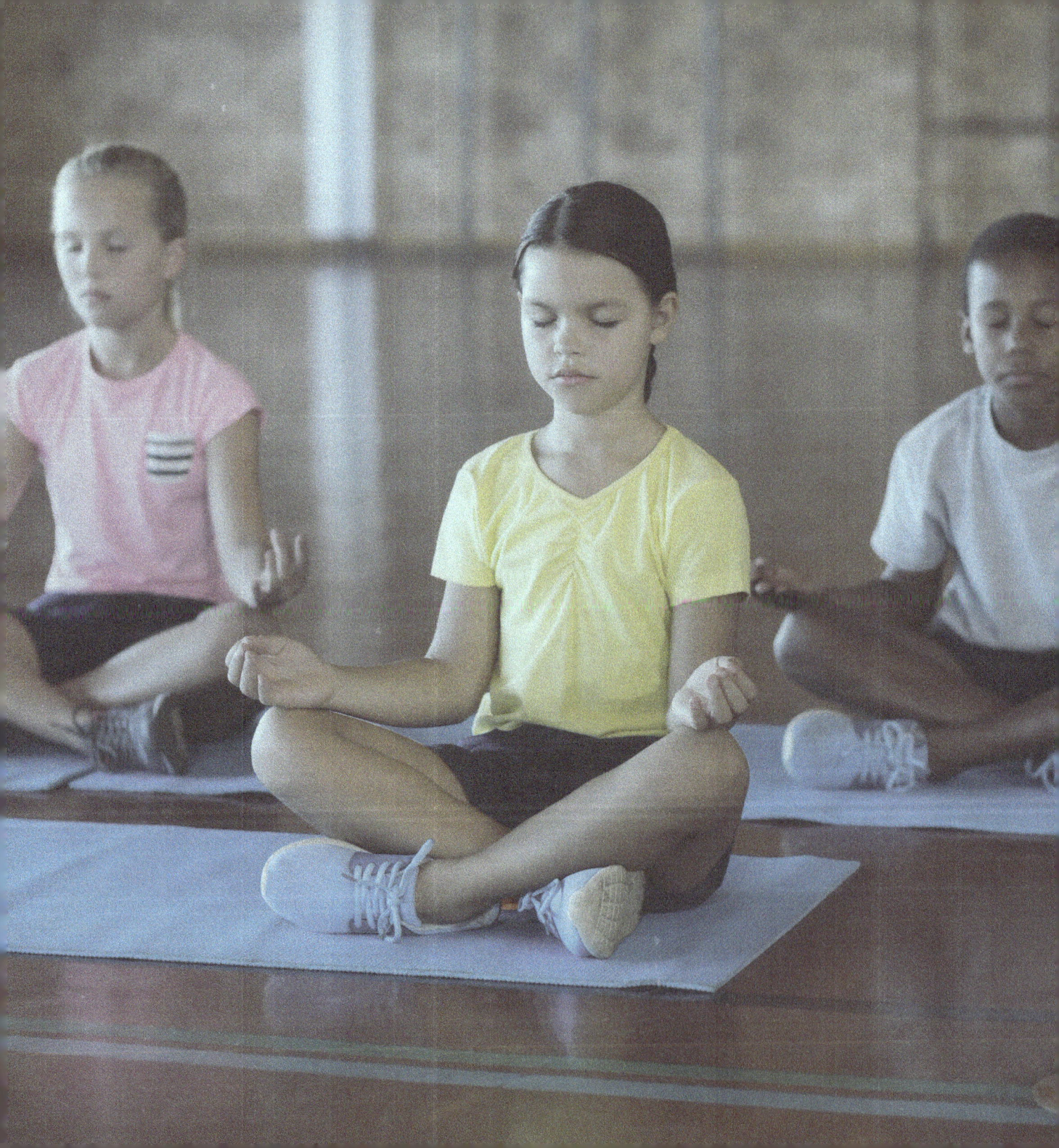

Stage 4

Go within:
why reclaiming life starts with mindfulness

> *On life's journey faith is nourishment, virtuous deeds are a shelter, wisdom is the light by day and right mindfulness is the protection by night. If a man lives a pure life, nothing can destroy him.*
>
> Buddha, spiritual leader, born as Siddhartha Gautama (ca.450 BCE–370 BCE)

Mindfulness can be defined as the quality, or state, of being conscious or aware of something. It is a mental state achieved by focusing attention on the present moment, while calmly acknowledging and accepting the feelings, thoughts and sensations at that moment. Today mindfulness is used as a therapeutic technique; however, mindful practices are part of every ancient wisdom tradition, including yoga and Buddhism. Used to calm and focus the mind, mindfulness helps us to focus on, and be in, the now, even in difficult situations.

In this stage, we will:

- Discuss the connection between body and mind, specifically looking at how our emotions impact on our physical health and can help us break the cycle of obesity.
- Identify and learn mindful practices, such as mindful eating, that help manage your emotions and your child's emotions around food.

What is mindfulness?

While it's beyond this book to provide a detailed approach to mindfulness, I want to introduce the concept to you. I strongly believe bringing some form of mindful attention to every aspect of your life, particularly while you are eating, is essential if you want to break the cycle of obesity in your family.

There is research to show the connection between body and mind, and it's helpful to understand how this applies to breaking the cycle of obesity. When you understand the connection, I am hopeful you will feel more compelled to take on board one or two simple mindful practices. My experience of these practices is that they're like the glue holding the other important physical actions in place.

What does mindfulness have to do with food?

Apart from nourishing us, food provides comfort too. If we consider the importance of food in and around religious and cultural festivals, such as Christmas, Passover, or after Ramadan, or as in my family at Chinese New Year, it's clear food has a special place in celebrations too.

When sourced, prepared and consumed in a balanced way, food is a wonderful thing. Unfortunately, for many people, eating food for comfort is taken to the extreme, along with other extreme behaviours around sourcing and preparing it. Instead of deriving nourishment and satisfying fulfilment, for many people living with obesity the consumption of food is a daily ritual of unhealthy food choices and thoughtless or mindless overeating and then guilt afterwards for overindulging.

When consumed in this manner, food is meeting unhealthy emotional needs. Rather than address underlying emotional issues, a person may continue to use food as a crutch because it's too painful or too hard to face the reality of the underlying cause (which could be one or many things). In many cases, the person is not aware of, or can't face, the root cause of this emotional overeating. If continued over a prolonged period, the outcomes can be dire, presenting as chronic disease, physical disability and, in the extreme, even death.

For other people, there are cultural challenges around food. In many cultures, food is considered as an expression of love and prosperity. (I know as I was brought up attending many Chinese banquets!) Often people feel the need to show love to their adult children and grandchildren through preparing excessive amounts of food. With many family gatherings characterised by large portion sizes and excessive volumes of food, it can be very difficult to step outside the unspoken cultural practice of overeating. Not discounting the health benefits to be gained from these cultural diets, the volume of food is far from healthy. The practice of pressuring others to eat more than they need or want is just as unhealthy as the eating itself, as is the agreement to eat when you don't want to (saying 'yes', when you really want to say 'no' – see stage 9 on the power of saying 'no').

Family Story

The grandparent effect: food as love

Jordan the Spider-Man boy is a delightful three-year-old old client of mine from a mixed ethnic family with food-loving Italian grandparents on one side and a Fijian–Chinese background on the other.

Jordan's mother is Italian and his father Fijian and both parents worked fulltime, so Jordan and his younger sister were looked after by one or other of his grandparents during the daytime. Food, especially processed foods, sweets and sugary drinks, was the way the grandparents expressed their love to their grandchildren.

This unhealthy intake of processed fake foods led to Jordan gaining excessive weight, so by the time he was three years of age he weighed almost 27kg.

I saw Jordan and his parents once and within three months Jordan starting eating 'power vegetables' as he kept saying to his parents after his first visit to see me. 'Dr Koala said I will be strong if I eat my veggies,' Jordan said, as he flexed his biceps eating carrots and cucumbers.

Both Jordan's mother and father had major concerns about the health of their children from eating so poorly when with their grandparents. When these concerns went unheeded, Jordan's mother decided as it was so stressful leaving her children with the grandparents, that she would reduce her work hours to take more direct care of them. She understood that this might be taken as a criticism of the grandparents but both grandfathers are now being more supportive and reminding their respective wives how important a healthier approach to food is. Giving the grandparents a copy of the growth chart depicting how far Jordan's weight was above even the top normal child's weight helped crystallise how abnormal the situation was and how important it was that changes were made.

Three months later, the family's stress level fell. Jordan's mother's stress in particular decreased significantly. Jordan's weight stabilised. In fact he lost 200g and grew over 2cm taller so his BMI dropped dramatically. I encouraged both parents to continue their courageous actions for their children's health and fully expect that this beautiful family will continue a healthier journey.

Jordan's mum's words:

Jordan was born at 4.95kg and continued to grow excessively over the next few years. We (me and my husband) were constantly being told that Jordan was a 'big boy', not only by our family and friends but also strangers. Despite this, we were passing what we had both grown up with on to him – lots of love and lots of food. We told ourselves it was in our genes and he would always be bigger than most people his age.

After seeing Dr Gary Leong, something clicked. I realised the severity of Jordan's weight gain and the possible health implications in the future. I didn't want to cause my son any harm, and it dawned on me that this is exactly what the whole extended family were doing in offering him poor food choices. In the next few weeks after we saw Dr Leong, Jordan started talking about Dr Koala more and more – saying he needed to eat his cucumbers and carrots to be strong like Spider-Man, as Dr Koala had said. Those cucumbers and carrots slowly turned Jordan into being open to trying and eating more fruit and veggies and he now eats very well for an active three-year-old! The whole family is now on board and I personally can feel the benefits of a healthier diet (clearer skin, more energy etc.).

Family Story

Marvellous Marval moving more

Marval was the fourth child of two busy parents in a Filipino family. Mum was working and studying commercial nutrition at TAFE and working long hours, sometimes night shifts while Dad was a lecturer at university, so both were well-educated parents. The care of this three-year-old boy was therefore largely left to his paternal grandmother who again loved to feed her grandson processed foods, sweets, juice and Yakult yoghurt drinks. The family had continued giving him baby formula in a bottle at night to try to get him to sleep.

He gained so much weight so by age three years he was 37kg. It became impossible for him to be carried by his mother and his father could carry him only with great difficulty. He could barely walk, only with great effort. Though he did not appear to have sleep apnoea, his large chest weight placed him at great risk of sleep apnoea.

Due to his weight he became very inactive. Being pushed around in a pram further aggravating any benefit of physical activity to slow down his weight gain. Instead he played and watched his iPad for hours to be entertained!

He had the dark rash on his neck called *acanthosis nigricans* confirming he had insulin resistance, the first step towards developing pre-diabetes and eventually type 2 diabetes, and often also associated with fatty liver disease. With encouragement and engagement of the grandmother and both parents, changes in his nutrition were made so he was able to slowly lose some weight. After six months there were still ongoing challenges as he was still being given Yakult and baby formula bottles at night increasing his risk of dental cavities and adding unnecessary calories to his diet.

We encouraged the parents to talk further with the grandmother to stop the Yakult, just give water at night, one normal cow's milk bottle during the day, to offer him more fresh vegetable snacks (carrots, cucumbers), smaller portions, avoid packaged snacks (chips and lollies) and try to get him more active with swimming lessons, walking and play group.

I have continued to follow this family as they have gained insight into how important these changes are for their son's long-term health, especially as there is a high risk of type 2 diabetes in the family. Change is difficult for most people and families, but these younger families highlight that it is better to make these changes in pre-school aged children, as it is so much more difficult later in childhood and especially once children reach the tricky teenage years!

How much of your eating is emotional?

As the Western diet of highly refined and high-sugar foods has infiltrated across the globe, there has been a corresponding deterioration in general health, presenting most obviously in the prevalence of obesity, which has doubled in more than 70 countries since 1980. What is most concerning is that during this period, the rate of increase in children was higher than for adults.[10] Alarm bells should be ringing everywhere.

All of this is serious stuff, but what does it have to do with you and mindfulness and food? Well, to answer that question, we need to ask another question, and it's a tough one.

Think about it this way: in response to stress, or feeling emotionally upset, do you automatically (mindlessly/without thinking) go to the pantry or fridge to find comfort in food? If your answer to this question is yes, it's time to get honest. It's also time to look for healthier ways to soothe yourself. When you gain control of this habit, you have a chance to help your child overcome this challenge too.

If you are using food for comfort, it's possible (even likely) that other members of your family are doing it too. Rest assured this is not a judgement. Rather, I'm raising this now because mindless eating – i.e. without thinking about what you eat, when you eat, and how fast you eat – is one of the core issues to address in breaking the cycle of obesity.

Identifying negative emotions and reactions

In stage 3, we talked about 'hooks' that trigger unhealthy behaviour. For many people, eating is habitual and ingrained as a way to feel better. We eat for a variety of reasons, not all of them to nourish us. For example, if you've had a bad day at work, you may be looking forward to a block of chocolate to help you feel better. If the kids have been driving you mad and your partner is out, you may be thinking of ordering takeaway as a treat to eat by yourself.

Now it's time to think carefully about your own emotions and behaviour. This exercise may elicit strong feelings. It is not an exercise designed to make you feel bad about yourself. It's about highlighting behaviours that may be keeping you from making healthier choices.

Can you identify one or two emotional reasons or situations that trigger a negative response in you, and record your usual response?

Emotion/situation	Response
1:	
2:	
3:	

Dealing with feelings around food

If completing the exercise above or any of the exercises in this book elicited strong emotions from you, you may wish to work through these feelings with a professional. There is no shame in asking for help. Talking to your GP, a counsellor or psychologist could help you to heal from past wounds and move forward to a healthier life.

With that in mind, let's look at your current approach to meals and food.

Common eating difficulties and problematic eating behaviours

- Food fighting: if a child refuses to eat a healthy nutritious meal you have prepared for dinner, then as per Ellyn Satter's Division of Responsibility, it is essential your child understands that it is your job or responsibility as a loving parent to decide what the child will eat and your child's decision whether to eat it or not. So do not compromise and give in to poor habits and processed packaged foods which continues the obesity cycle. Change is difficult but leading by example as a parent and your persistence will be rewarded.
- Food refusal: Again as per food fighting refusing to eat is a behaviour common to children with obesity. However by giving your child the opportunity to decide whether he or she will eat what you have prepared or go hungry is their choice. Trying again through your healthy example is the only way to proceed.
- Binge eating: this is a very difficult problem to overcome but focusing on mindfulness and mindful eating of real living nutritious food is they key to start changing this abnormal relationship with food.

- Food bribery: by using food (especially unhealthy snacks and drinks) as a reward one sets up unhealthy obsession with processed food as a way parents influence behaviour. Use non-food retreads for positive behaviour is the way to go.
- Refusal to eat in public, including at school: A common behaviour is the adolescent girl, but sometimes boy, refusing to eat in public. This often leads to missed lunch at school and leaves the child unhealthily and ravishingly hungry when school is finished, causing binge overeating of the wrong foods which perpetuates the whole cycle.
- Secret eating: Sadly, sneaking food is common in some children as they cannot be sated by eating processed, high-calorie, sugary foods. This is opposed to the nutritious, real rainbow- coloured fruit and vegetables and good quality protein and fats that are all part of the mindful, slow, healthy eating plan I advocate.

Eating mindfully

Eating mindfully starts well before you sit down to a meal.

It starts in the planning, and then the preparation of the family meal.

You need to take this mindfulness to the shop when you buy the groceries for the meal to avoid straying from the shopping list. Mindfulness is also needed when preparing the meal, setting the table, eating the meal and in the clean up afterwards.

Approaching your food and eating in this way may seem onerous, but you will be surprised once you start these practices how different your response to food is, and how your relationship with food changes for the better. It will be the same for your kids too.

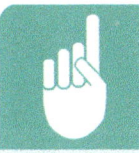
Just One Thing rule

Apply the **Just One Thing** rule to a single mindful action you can take with respect to food. Try doing this one thing every time you sit to eat. It could be as simple as:
- Taking three deep slow breaths before you start eating
- Chopping the ingredients for the meal more slowly
- Taking time to look at and smell what's on your plate before starting your meal
- Savouring and chewing each mouthful of food
- Eating shared meals around a dining table with no distractions (including television and phones)
- Being thankful for your food by expressing gratitude for the meal and life generally.

Encourage other family members to do the same and observe how your appreciation of food changes.

Mealtimes

What's the environment like in which you share your meals? You may be surprised to know that how you eat has a significant impact on the way in which food is consumed.

Does your family eat meals together at a dining table without distractions like smartphones, iPads and televisions? Or does everyone eat at different times and locations, without any conversation or connection?

Is there stress at mealtimes? Are there arguments at the dinner table? Equally, are there silent tensions that make mealtimes uncomfortable?

Create a healthy environment for meals

One of the first ways you can create change is by establishing a stable and consistent environment for eating meals mindfully. The very best way to do this is by sitting at the table together as a family at a regular time each day. This is one of the iron-clad rules I emphasise with my patients and their families.

To do this, you need a dining table. If you don't have a table at which your family can share a meal, you need to get one. It's that simple. A fundamental tool for implementing change, a dining table is where the action happens. It doesn't need to be brand new, expensive or special; you just need one. An inexpensive, functional table can be sourced secondhand, online, or even from a family member or friend who perhaps wishes to declutter their own home!

Once you have your table, it also needs be clear of junk and used solely for the purpose of the family sharing meals together. In breaking the cycle of obesity, your dining table is a sacred space in your family's home.

If this is new behaviour for your family, it is essential to communicate the new state of play clearly about the need for the new behaviour and how it's going happen practically. You will also need to specify the role each family member has to contribute to the new way of doing things.

Explain to each member of your family the importance of eating together around the family table as many nights a week as possible. There can be no excuses for one child going off to their room and being isolated. So one has to be firm that dinner is at a set time and everyone is expected to be there prior to that time to help set the table and provide any help to get the meal ready. If an adolescent initially refuses and goes off in a temper tantrum to their room then that is fine but do not allow them to eat if they do not wish to be part of this essential new family rule. They will soon enough smell the beautiful food you have prepared and their hunger will eventually bring them out of their shell.

I know parents have different timetables but this same rule should apply for both parents who know they have to be home at a certain time for dinner.

Once this habit is established, I see so many families become transformed and who start to love this family time together and feel this allows them time to connect, communicate and contribute to being part of their special family.

How to share a mindful meal together

There is sitting at the table together but being disconnected, and there is sitting at the table together in a mindful way. Mindful eating together as a family looks like this:

- All members of the family at the table together at an agreed, regular, non-negotiable time of the evening.
- There is a shared appreciation of the meal and preparation taken to bring it to the table.
- There is NO technology at the table or in the room. Television and phones are switched off (no exceptions – it's a non-negotiable).
- There are no phones at the table. If necessary, provide a basket for everyone to put their phones in before sitting down and place the basket away from the table. No exceptions – it's a non-negotiable for every single meal.

- Everyone stays at the table for the duration of the meal – a balanced, mindful meal experience requires 30 minutes of time, making it an ideal opportunity to connect and catch up with one another through deeper communication enabled by conversation, celebration of wins, expression of concerns, and looking ahead.
- If you find it challenging to have conversations around the dinner table, then please see the exercise below on how to do this.
- Before you embark on your new dinner routine, discuss as a family the expectation of politeness and respect at the table.
- Each family member paces their eating without rushing, taking at least 20 minutes to consume a healthy meal size.
- Finally try to eat until you are satisfied or comfortably full, not uncomfortably full. I use a hunger Emoji scale card to help kids and their families train themselves to try to get in tune with their physical feelings of hunger before the meal, feelings of becoming full during the meal and satiation after the end of their meal (see foodinsight.org/learn-how-to-eat-mindfully-with-the-eat-mojis-infographic/).

When you start the process of creating new habits around meals, the established patterns of eating will become more apparent to you. You may notice a child with obesity will probably eat quickly, while a child who is not overweight, but fussy, may take much longer to finish their meal, if allowed. Resist the temptation to be negative and criticise your child's eating habits. Rather, this is where it's important for the parent to be the leader and demonstrate where change needs to occur. Fast, mindless eaters must learn to pace themselves and finish their meal more slowly and mindfully, i.e. taking between 20 to 30 minutes to eat.

Conversation starters

If having conversations at the dinner table is a relatively new concept for your family, you might like to try this as a means of introducing the idea. Make each person responsible for bringing a new topic for discussion to the table each day. For example, encourage that person to read a snippet out of a book, news item, or something the teacher was talking about at school. It could be something that starts with: 'Did you know that...' or 'In some countries they do...'

Each person also has to share one thing they learned that day. And it can be anything at all. You can even make this a funny part of the conversation. For example, I learned today that cats really do like to chase mice, but none of them are really called Jerry.

The other part of this is to give everyone a chance to speak. You may start by going around the table, each day someone else gets to start first, and asking these simple questions of everyone: What was the best part of your day? What made it so?

In time these questions will become easy and fun, and you might learn some interesting things about each other and the world in general. Sometimes you may also find that the conversation extends well past dinner and on into the evening.

There are also card packs you can buy with 'conversation starters' on them. You can draw a card for each evening meal and go from there.

When you are eating a meal and exploring conversation, you also eat slower and more mindfully as you go. One of the rules being that, when it's your turn to speak, you have to put your knife and fork down for the moment.

Establishing a new routine around mealtimes will help you and your family redefine a new and healthier relationship with food. Food becomes nourishing as do the family relationships, which are strengthened through these mealtime connections.

Building resilience

As I've already stated, it's important to integrate changes slowly.

Approach the establishment of these mindful eating habits in a manageable and sustainable way, by taking small steps. If you hope to break the cycle of obesity for life, holding firm to the new rules around mindful meals, there needs to be no compromise. To do this, you need to be resilient. The way to build that resilience is to:

- **Remember your why for breaking the cycle of obesity.** It's not an exaggeration to say the lives of your children depend on you holding strong to your why. Remember you are giving them the gift of life and that makes holding firm to boundaries worthwhile.
- **Take very good care of yourself.** It is only when you feel emotionally stable and strong that you'll be able to overcome the resistance that arises when you're embedding new behaviours.

Try not to lose heart if not all family members are as enthusiastic and agreeable to the changes you're initiating. Human nature is such that people resist change, even if it's good, and often the greatest resistance comes just before acceptance. Once you have established a new routine – which typically might take a month to become habitual – and it is apparent you're steadfast in your intent, you'll have created a ripple effect that eventually leads each person in the family to make a decision. They'll decide whether they're in or out, i.e. choose a healthier, happier life or continue on a pathway that takes away life. A difference in choice (healthy versus unhealthy) is not an excuse for you to prepare multiple meals to suit the specific tastes of every family member. It's one nutritious meal for all – remember, it's one rule for all.

In the family, you the parent are responsible for providing the food and your child is responsible for eating it. So if your teenager decides she doesn't like chicken and vegetables, they can go without dinner. It's up to you to allow them the space to make that decision and accept the consequences that go with it, including continued weight gain and the feelings associated with that.

Family Story

Teenage mindful vs mindless eating battles

Susan, at two years old was always hungry; she never felt full after eating. This led Susan to develop a 'vacuum-cleaner' eating style, as her father described it to me.

Both parents were obese and there was a strong family history of type 2 diabetes, mellitus and heart disease on both sides of the family. As a teenager, Susan would finish her meals in five to 10 minutes and although she had eaten enough to be full, she was still hungry so kept eating till she felt 'stuffed'!

The family struggled with Susan's unhealthy relationship with food. Consuming large portions and snacking on processed foods (which were available in the pantry and house) she progressively gained excessive weight throughout her childhood. Despite being a black belt in jujitsu and doing well at school, at 14 and a half years of age she was 114.2kg, and her BMI was 45.6kg/m^2 with a waist circumference of 132cm.

She had clinical and blood evidence of insulin resistance but did not have pre-diabetes or diabetes, though she was at high risk of developing diabetes in the following five years unless her weight gain could be reversed. She was on maximum dose of metformin 2g/day to reduce her insulin resistance. She had no clinical signs of polycystic ovarian disease (PCOS) as she had no evidence of excessive hair growth or irregular menstrual periods.

We focused on trying to help the whole family eat more slowly and more mindfully so that she developed an awareness when she had eaten enough to be satisfied rather than being overly full.

I saw her for a year and the family also sought the help of a private dietitian. The family also completed their kitchen renovation and started to eat together around their new dining table at dinner time. This helped Susan and her whole family to eat smaller portions, slower and more mindfully. Despite these significant changes Susan still continued to gain weight albeit less than before. Her weight rose to 119.1 kg and her BMI rose to $48kg/m^2$. When Susan and her mother started a very low energy diet (VLED), they consumed meal-replacement shakes for breakfast and healthy portions of protein and salads and vegetables for lunch and dinner. They followed ketotic diet (low carbohydrate intake) and drank lots of water while maintaining good levels of physical activity (jujitsu). Susan also went to the gym with a close friend a few times a week.

However, after several months and sessions with a clinical psychologist and dietitian, Susan was unable to find the inner motivation to sustain these changes. While her mother lost significant weight on VLED, Susan continued to gain weight up to 123kg which set up some discord and stress between her and her mother. Susan continued to be unable to moderate her food intake as she worked part-time in a fast-food restaurant. She has not been able to overcome her hunger drive. Stress at the demands of senior high school also continued to fuel her emotional overeating.

Sometimes until an adolescent has the internally driven motivation to change, their struggle continues. Not until the young person develops new relationships and peers (sometimes away from the parental influence) or a new work or vocational or study opportunity arises will the adolescent then come under the effect of healthier social networks that prioritise healthier eating and a more physically active and mindful life.

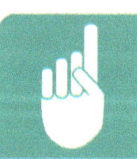

A word about relationships and changes

If your partner chooses not to support your decision for healthier meals, and a more mindful approach to their eating, be aware it may lead to significant tension in this relationship. A decision to improve your health – yours and your child's – may open cracks in your relationship with your partner that haven't been addressed previously. Despite this, please do not allow it to deflect you from your chosen path for you and your child. Additional suggestions for how to manage these challenging situations are presented in stage 9; The power of 'no'.

Mindful practices around food and meals

Bringing mindfulness to mealtimes doesn't mean you turn yourself into a Buddhist monk. However, it does mean you bring some simple mindful practices to your food and meals. I've developed my own techniques that I've seen work when applied consistently.

- **Always 'taste with your face'.** A term coined by Dr George and Penny Blair-West, 'taste with your face' means using all your senses during preparation and eating of meals.[11] Rather than rushing through a meal, tasting with your face allows you to take time to savour the flavours, textures and joy a meal provides. Approaching meals this way slows our eating down; by the nature of savouring things, you must eat slower. A direct consequence is you eat less whilst enjoying your meal more, because you're satisfied and aware that you're satisfied. Bonus!
- **Let your child feed themselves.** For the young child who is old enough to cut their own food and feed themselves, allow them to do this. By taking the responsibility for this aspect of their mealtime, they will be forced to slow down their eating. As long as you have shown them the correct way to cut their food and eat it (remembering you will need to do this many times), using the 'taste with your face' approach, you will be on the road to establishing a new mindful practice around food that will change their whole life. What a gift!
- **Hands-free eating.** In the clinic, I tell my patients to let go of the eating utensils in between mouthfuls of food to avoid the typical 'vacuum suctioning' style of food consumption. Instead, concentrate on chewing the food well. Important for slowing down the eating process, chewing more thoroughly has many benefits for the rest of the digestive process. Well-chewed food is more easily metabolised by the body, allowing the hormonal signals to the brain to activate the centre that regulates whether a person feels satisfied or not. It also allows your body to extract the nourishment from the food that isn't possible when you eat very quickly, without chewing properly. In between mouthfuls of food, you can engage in and stimulate healthy conversation around the table. Together, these factors create the possibility of better connection – with yourself and the family.
- **Eat more real food.** Include more real food in your meals, and make it rainbow coloured. I'm not talking about unicorns here. Rather I am referring to the glorious colours of the

real, living, natural food that is available to all Australians at their local grocer or fruit and veggie market. We are living in a country abounding in beautiful food sources, so use them! Explore what good-value markets are around your neighbourhood or support or contribute to a local community garden (www.cityofsydney.nsw.gov.au/community/participation/community-gardens or www.communitygarden.org.au). Or be bold and consider growing some of your own food, especially vegetables such as tomatoes or herbs (www.localharvest.org.au/learn/a-quick-guide-to-growing-your-own-food).

- **Smaller plate, smaller portion.** Part of the epidemic of global obesity is the growing plate and portion size that has contributed to the corresponding expansion in waistlines. In simple terms, this means putting less on the plate. As the old saying goes, less is more: healthy, nutritious, satisfying food that is eaten more slowly. See stage 5 for more information on portion sizes.
- **Smile while you eat.** When we eat mindlessly, the last thing we do is smile. As we become more mindful during meals, we can pause and reflect and yes, we can smile too. A smile indicates we're enjoying our food and the experience of sharing our meal with family. The other thing about smiles is they're contagious. Once you start smiling at the table, you may be surprised by the realisation of how little you have smiled during meals. This awareness is intended to bring more mindfulness to your meals.
- **Drink a glass of water during dinner.** There are differing opinions among experts about the merits of drinking water at mealtimes. However, I am an advocate of this practice. It is clear most people do not drink adequate amounts of water during the day, and when thirsty, they drink sugar-sweetened beverages, which contribute to the cycle of obesity. Ban all sugar drinks at the table and instead stick with just cold water, as cold water quenches thirst more effectively than room-temperature water.

When you become successful at applying mindfulness to your food, eating and drinking, you will discover it can be applied to other aspects of your life. It will enhance and nourish you, bringing improvements to your mental and physical health.

Resources

Make sure you also get across to the Ride to Life website and access all the online resources that are available there.

For some of the best mindful eating resources available I highly recommend those of Dr Susan Albers, a clinical psychologist from Cleveland Clinic in the USA.

Susan has written numerous helpful books on mindful eating, including one for adolescents called *Eating Mindfully for Teens*. Susan also has great free on-line resources at www.eatingmindfully.com, so start working on that 20–30 minute rule and reclaim the 'Joy' from your food.

Jean Hailes for Women's Health – Mindful eating poster tip sheet at: assets.jeanhailes.org.au/Mindful_eating_poster.pdf

The Foundation for a Mindful Society, USA at www.mindful.org/6-ways-practice-mindful-eating/

Yoga Journal: an excellent on-line resource for yoga and mindfulness at www.yogajournal.com/

The official BKS Iyengar yoga website at bksiyengar.com/

Iyengar yoga Australia at iyengaryoga.asn.au/

Yoga International online teaching and resources: yogainternational.com/

Taste with Your Face – Adventures in Healthy Eating: a children's book by Dr George and Penny Blair-West, adult psychiatrist and psychologist. Available through online bookstores.

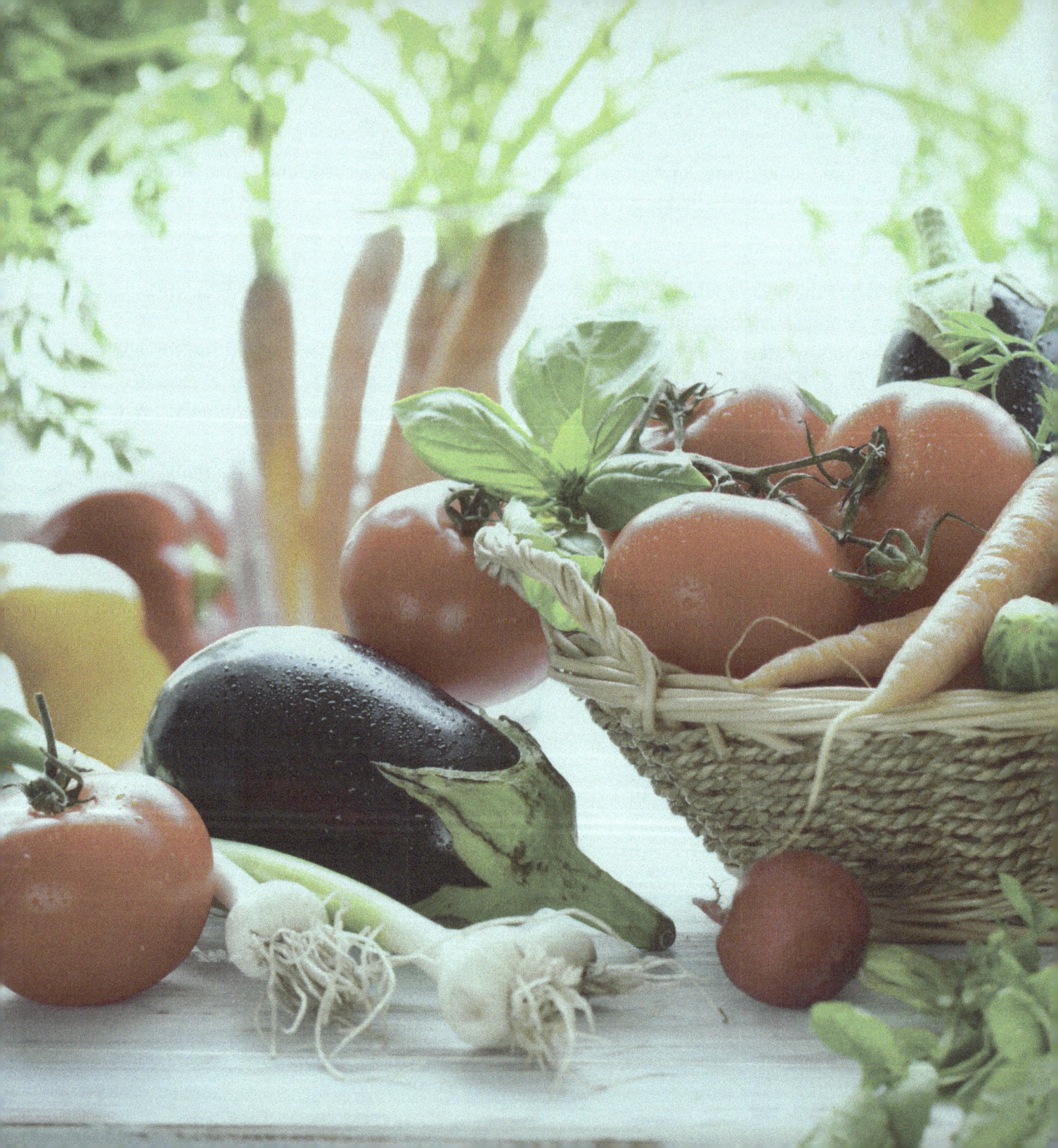

Stage 5

You are what you eat: nutrition for making the change for good

> *Let food be thy medicine and medicine be thy food*
>
> Hippocrates, Ancient Greek physician of Age of Pericles 460BCE–377BCE, regarded as father of practice of medicine as a rational science

A mountain (or two) of books has been written about nutrition and what constitutes a healthy diet and it is not my intention to add to it. What I do want to do is provide practical information you can apply to your own set of circumstances.

In this stage, we:

- Outline the principles of good nutrition.
- Start the journey to developing the skills needed to prepare healthy meals at home.

Principles of good nutrition

When I start working with patients on this aspect, I ask a simple question. If your grandparents saw the food you eat, would they recognise it as the real, living food they ate when they were children?

I ask this question because in the time before the globalisation of fast-food brands like McDonald's, KFC, Pizza Hut and Hungry Jacks, takeaway or fast food was only available in a very limited way, if at all. Almost everybody prepared fresh food at home, and while this food may have been simple – meat and three vegetables – meals were nourishing, healthy and in no way super-sized. Reflected in the physical size of people and their physique – generally lean and physically fit – food was regarded as sustenance, not something for self-soothing.

In the same way, hunger was considered a normal daily sensation felt between main meals. Sweets were in short supply and baked at home from real ingredients. Often grown at home, fruit and vegetables formed an essential part of the normal daily diet. People knew where their food came from. Parents decided what would go on the table (i.e. they weren't dictated to by kids), and children ate their food without complaint or if they did complain, parents generally ignored them. That was the way I was brought up. On special occasions (and there were always enough of those during the year to satisfy most kids), but not every day, my parents allowed us to indulge in a special ice cream or sweet, which we enjoyed more as we knew it was a special occasion!

The principles of nutrition during that era were simple. I feel very strongly that these principles have become overcomplicated as knowledge has grown; although ironically, the increased knowledge about food hasn't kept us healthy – remember the prevalence of obesity statistics I quoted in the introduction?

There is so much nutritional information available, but much of it is conflicting and confusing. I can understand why families struggling with obesity feel overwhelmed. It seems like every week there's a new diet or superfood to get on board with. The reality is every diet will find people for whom it works incredibly well. Some people will get onto the paleo or keto diet and lose the weight they've always wanted to. Other people will eat a low-fat diet and get healthy. Some people will stick to a low-GI diet and reap the rewards of good health.

As someone who treats patients with obesity each day, I feel that people who are committed to breaking the cycle of obesity in their family need to go back to basic principles. And that's what I'm going to share here in this book. These basic principles will provide a framework within which you can find what works for you and your family. Once you're confident in these principles, you may wish to experiment, but for now, simple is best.

Time to build confidence in your food wisdom

To reconnect with yourself, establish a healthy relationship with food, and break the cycle of obesity, you must find what works best for you and your family. This means slowing down enough to allow you to tune in and observe your family's needs.

Yes, we need to receive guidance about relevant nutritional information about eating in a balanced and healthy way. We also need to take that information and configure it for our own set of circumstances. Although it may take time to build this food wisdom 'muscle', it's important to understand this is the direction you'll be moving in. Ultimately, it comes down to taking full responsibility for your own health and wellbeing, which is really what's at the heart of breaking the cycle of obesity.

One important step in the process of building your food wisdom muscle is to recognise there is no 'one size fits all' food regimen. Part of breaking the cycle of obesity means you are also on a journey of discovery of food that gives life and vitality to your family. Having said that, I believe there are principles which create sensible food foundations for every person. Within the family unit there may be individual preferences, but there is going to be a large area of overlap that allows you to cater to most people's needs most of the time and to do this in a healthy way.

Remember, I'm not a diet dictator. I'm simply sharing the guiding principles I apply and know work for patients in my clinic.

Dr Gary's four simple food tips for breaking the cycle of obesity

1. Substitute empty, fake, fast foods for nourishing, real wholefoods – so-called 'rainbow' fresh foods, i.e. fresh fruit and vegetables, lentils, wholegrains and whole foods.
2. Keep food simple and unprocessed.
3. Incorporate as much plant food as possible into your diet.
4. Moderate meal sizes at home and when eating out.

That's it.

Now you might be reading this and thinking, *Come on, Gary. I need more than that. I need details.* I can assure you we'll get to that, but in its essence, what I advocate to patients is they adopt these principles and 'work' them like their lives depend on them. In many respects, they do.

Without wanting to simplify things too much, I subscribe to the philosophy that simple is best. It's unhelpful to get on the bandwagon of every fad and diet. It's no mistake diet books are one of the most popular genres of books sold. This is only because people want a quick fix without facing the underlying emotional and socio-cultural issues that have caused them to be caught up in the cycle of obesity and being unhealthily overweight.

Ride to Life is not one of those books. I have said many times already – and I'll continue to repeat it – there is no quick fix for an individual with obesity, only small, steady steps towards sustainable change.

In the same vein, eating whole, healthy foods rather than processed foods is best for you, as is the inclusion of as much plant food as possible. I expand on these ideas below, but if you take nothing else out of this book and just approach your food in this way I am confident you will start seeing visible and positives differences in your health and your family's health.

Sizing your meals right is vital too. There is a direct correlation between growth in waistlines and the size of meals, so aiming to reduce meal sizes is important. I have also included additional principles below, which I encourage my patients to adopt. As with other aspects of the healthy keys to breaking the cycle of obesity, I recommend you start with one principle and work at integrating this slowly into your daily life. For example, start with breakfast, get that right, and then move to the next area of focus.

Eat breakfast every day

No doubt you've heard you should eat a healthy breakfast. Contrary to what you may think, this is not some old wives' tale. As life has become busier, people have struggled with maintaining important routines. Breakfast, along with many other stabilising practices, has fallen by the wayside. If that's the case in your family, then now is the time to get back on that bandwagon.

It is so important you and your child have a healthy breakfast together, if possible, every day. Without appropriate fuel to kickstart the day, your child is already on the back foot. After an overnight fast, the body requires healthy energy to awaken and fuel the brain and body to be ready to learn and be active. The real benefits of breakfast are not always visible to the naked eye; however, you will notice the difference when they present as:

- Improved concentration and short-term memory
- Increased likelihood your child will maintain a healthy weight due to reduced snacking
- Improved focus in the classroom
- Improved behaviour from eating a balanced meal
- Better maintenance of blood sugar and hormone levels.

When I see people in my clinic, they feel very confused about what makes a healthy breakfast. This is understandable because we are constantly bombarded with marketing from food companies that dress up breakfast products as healthy for kids. I know I've said I'm not dictatorial when it comes to food, but there is one exception: I'm absolutely against the marketing of empty foods as healthy.

Turn on any television or walk into any supermarket and you won't miss it – the deluge of false advertising designed to tempt you and your family into buying food that is nutritionally empty. This is why I tell parents, you must be aware that you are entering a battle zone when you go to the supermarket! If you walk down the middle aisles of any large chain supermarket looking for healthy options, you will be disappointed. And guess where the breakfast cereals are located? The middle aisles!

As you get further along your journey, you will start to recognise the signs that indicate where particular products and foods are not healthy. Most packaged breakfast cereals are high in refined sugar and have no place at your family's breakfast table. The only cereals I recommend to patients are rolled oats, Weet-Bix or comparable gluten-free alternatives, such as rolled rice.

Good options for a healthy breakfast include:

- Weet-Bix with banana and milk
- Steel-cut oats soaked overnight with dates or mixed berries
- Poached or boiled eggs on wholegrain or sourdough toast
- Fruit salad with natural (unsweetened) yoghurt
- Untoasted muesli with milk
- A slice of multigrain toast with nut butter and a glass of milk
- A homemade English muffin with a slice of ham, egg and cheese
- Omelette with ham and vegetables.

Breakfast for the time-poor

Mornings are often a frantic time for families. Depending on your hours of work, you may be up and out the door early without eating, thinking you'll 'get something on the way' and end up grabbing something unhealthy or not eating at all. I believe getting up slightly earlier and taking an extra ten minutes to eat together at the table is the ideal way to start the day. If you can sit down most mornings with your child and demonstrate a commitment to a healthy breakfast, that will set up a strong start to the day for everyone.

There may be times when work commitments or particularly busy weeks mean a sit-down breakfast is very difficult to achieve. If you are aware of an upcoming busy time, you can plan ahead to ensure you still get a nutritious breakfast.

Here are some ideas for making breakfast more efficient:

- Prepare rolled oats (organic steel-cut if you can find them) with yoghurt, milk and fruit the night before and leave them in the fridge. Come morning, just whip out your pre-made breakfast and you're good to go.
- Pack yourself an on-the-go breakfast the night before. A hard-boiled egg, a piece of fruit, a jar of oats and yoghurt and a bottle of water and you're all set.
- Set the table with cutlery, bowls and glasses the night before. Even a few minutes saved can make all the difference.
- Encourage all family members to rinse and stack their dishes once they have finished to contribute to the tidying-up process.

Eat balanced meals at lunch and dinner

One technique I use to explain the concept of a balanced meal with my patients is asking them to think of their dinner plate and split it into three sections. One quarter should be filled with a good-quality protein, one quarter with low-GI complex carbohydrates (we'll get to this shortly), and the remaining half of the plate should be filled with a variety of fresh vegetables (cooked and/or raw). Approach every meal in this balanced way, and you will soon start to see the benefits of your efforts.

Enjoy healthy snacks

Snacks are a great way to get all the nutrients to keep the body and brain functioning. However, snacks should be healthy, not the unhealthy packaged foods that fill supermarket and convenience store shelves.

Here are some suggestions to encourage your child to eat healthy snacks:

- Plan ahead by creating a day-to-day menu of what snacks your child is allowed to eat. Place this plan on the fridge so your child knows what they can have. When possible prepare and

store these items in the fridge or pantry so your child can simply grab them and go.
- To avoid temptation, remove processed snack foods from the household. As you prepare your shopping list, don't add these items to it. Remember, if it's not in the cupboard, you can't eat it. If it doesn't make it to the shopping trolley, it can't make it to the cupboard and into meals.
- Keep a selection of healthy snacks in the house such as milk, yoghurt, chopped fruit, nuts and wholegrain seeded bread.
- Think about serving sizes. Snacks are not meals and should not be too big. Instead they should only be large enough to keep your child satisfied until their next meal.
- Consider the timing of snacks. Do not allow children to become so hungry they want to eat everything in sight or overeat. Schedule snacks at regular times each day.
- Reflect on where snacks are consumed. Avoid eating in front of the television or computer where mindless eating occurs more easily.
- Be a healthy role model. Children will follow your example. Eating healthier snacks and offering to share them with your child is an effective way of subtly introducing new behaviours.
- Involve your child in the kitchen by creating snack packs together, for example mixing dried fruits and nuts in zip-lock bags or creating fruit kebabs.
- Get creative. Allow your child to experiment in the kitchen with new foods and flavours. When it comes to dried fruits, however, remember to think in terms of moderation. A few raisins or apricots is fine, but fresh is best I think as these contain less sugar.

Suggestions for healthy snacks include:

- A banana rolled in yoghurt, then rolled in crushed nuts and frozen
- Fingers of wholemeal toast with Vegemite (or an equivalent sugar-free spread)
- Hard-boiled eggs
- Carrot, cucumber, celery or capsicum sticks with healthy dips or cream cheese
- Plain unsweetened Greek yoghurt with mixed berries (frozen ones are fine)
- Cheese cubes
- Fresh fruit with plain, unsweetened Greek yoghurt – or homemade yoghurt, which is easy and quick to do actually if you know how, and can save you money!

Perfect your portion sizes

In a world where super-sized meals have become the norm, breaking the cycle of obesity means re-establishing a new healthy normal for portion sizes. Distorted portion sizes are a major reason for the modern cycle of obesity. We simply eat too much at every meal – and in between too! Hunger is now seen as an abnormal part of our daily existence. However, when I was growing up, my parents knew I'd be fine (even if I was briefly a little hungry) as they knew I would receive a healthy nutritious meal within a very short time. I say this to highlight how important hunger is before a main meal to regulate your child's appetite and eagerness to eat what's placed in front of them.

What about the child who's always hungry?

This is a common dilemma for parents who attend my clinic. They cannot stop their child from overeating because of this incredible drive to eat, despite the child eating portions that are well beyond what is appropriate for their age. I have found the children are acutely aware of the problem too. When I ask them about the 'Hunger Monsters', the kids always know what I'm referring to – a little mischievous smile on their beautiful faces betrays their little secret. The trick to helping with these seemingly insatiable Hunger Monsters is realising the food you're feeding your child is the root of the problem. This plus mindless fast eating (finishing your main meal like a 'vacuum cleaner', as some parents describe it to me) all contribute to a vicious hunger overeating cycle.

Dealing with the Hunger Monsters

The Hunger Monsters that drive your child's desperate need to eat and eat and eat arise from the effects of the artificial, fast and processed foods that contain highly refined carbohydrates, saturated fat and high levels of salt.

Eating unhealthy foods makes your child's blood sugar levels rise rapidly. In response, your child's pancreas releases a large spike of insulin, the hormone that lowers blood sugar. But then, typically, this rise in insulin causes a rapid drop in blood sugar, and then about an hour afterwards your child's brain responds with a hunger drive. Feeding this hungry drive with unhealthy food starts the process all over again: blood sugar rises, insulin is deployed to lower blood sugar which then leads to more hunger which is then fed with unhealthy food. This behaviour keeps them in the cycle of obesity.

It is the chronic intake of artificial processed food which leads to a permanent state of high insulin in the body. Eventually, this leads to a state of insulin resistance, which means the insulin hormone is no longer working with the body to keep it healthy. Instead, it is abnormally compensating for the obesity and abnormal weight distribution in the body, i.e. around the abdomen, within the liver and in the skeletal muscles of your child.

This insulin-resistance state, with its higher insulin levels, has a direct effect on the appetite centre within the brain. Leptin is our most important appetite-suppressing hormone and it is secreted from fat cells throughout the body. When leptin is suppressed by insulin, there is an unhealthy increase in appetite and hunger.

Breaking this vicious cycle of unnatural hunger and overeating requires that you and your family use the power of real, living, nutritious food to reset your child's brain's appetite-control centres. Professor David Ludwig has written an entire book on this devastating cycle. *Always Hungry? Conquer cravings, retrain your fat cells and lose weight permanently* describes how this cycle works in our bodies. It is well worth a read if you want to understand more of the science behind what is going on with your child.

Another stressful dimension to this cycle of fighting the Hunger Monsters is the emotions associated with the corresponding food fight between the parent and child. It is possible to stop the food fight,[12] but it does require you to change the food you feed your child. It also requires that you set and hold firm to new boundaries (more about this in stage 9). I acknowledge this is going to be difficult initially. In fact, expect it to get worse before it gets better. In many senses, it will be a withdrawal process and you can expect resistance from your child's body and their emotional and physical attachment to the unhealthy processed foods they have been accustomed to eating.

While these changes may not be accepted by your child overnight, in even a week, slowly but surely, this healthier eating will become the norm. Reassure them that you are doing this because you love them despite what they may say to you initially! To make these changes more acceptable, get your children involved in choosing new real food – e.g. vegetables and fruits to try – and definitely involve them in the preparation of the new healthy meals. As many parents have themselves lost the art of healthy, simple cooking, you may need help! Fortunately, there is a wealth of resources online and in books that teach you how to prepare simple, nutritious and cost-effective meals (see link to Ride to Life recipe resources and others including *Jamie's Ministry of Food* and *Simply Recipes*).

You are literally saving your child's life by taking this important step and choosing healthy, nourishing food over empty, 'nothing', fake food.

Standard serves

The Australian Government's Eat for Health guidelines for serve sizes is summarised in the table below and it shows the number of serves per food group for children between the ages of two and 18 years. Standard serve sizes can be confusing, which makes the detail provided around weight and kilojoule conversion very helpful. The serve size is a set amount that doesn't change but the number of serves equals the portion size.

Check out *Portion Perfection* from Amanda Clark (www.greatideas.net.au) which is a great real-life photo guide to healthy portions for children age four to 13 years. Trudy Williams is another pioneering dietician. Check out www.foodtalk.com.au/contents/en-us/about.html.

Food group	Example equivalent standard serves
Vegetables & legumes/beans A standard serve of vegetables is about 75g (100–350kJ)	• ½ cup cooked, dried or canned beans, peas or lentils • 1 cup green leafy or raw salad vegetables • ½ cup sweet corn • ½ medium potato or other starchy vegetables (sweet potato, taro or cassava) • 1 medium tomato
Fruit A standard serve of fruit is about 150g (350kJ)	• 1 medium apple, banana or pear • 2 small apricots, kiwi fruits or plums • 1 diced or canned fruit (with no added sugar) • 125ml juice (½ cup with no added sugar), occasionally • 30g dried fruit; for example, 4 dried apricot halves, 1½ tablespoons sultanas

Food group	Example equivalent standard serves
Grain (cereal) foods, mostly wholegrain A standard serve is 500kJ	- 1 slice (40g) of bread ½ medium (40g) roll or flat bread - ½ cup (75–100g) cooked rice, pasta, noodles, - ½ cup barley, buckwheat, semolina, polenta, bulgar, or quinoa - ½ cup (125g) cooked porridge - 3 (35g) crispbreads - 1 small English muffin or scone
Lean meats and poultry, fish, eggs, tofu, nuts, seeds A standard serve is 500–600kJ	- 65g lean meats such as beef, lamb, veal, pork, goat or kangaroo (approximately 90–100g raw) - 80g cooked lean poultry such as chicken or turkey (100g raw) - 100g cooked fish fillet (about 115g raw weight) or 1 small can of fish - 2 large eggs - 1 cup (150g) cooked or canned legumes/beans such as lentils, chickpeas or split peas (without salt) - 170g tofu - 30g nuts, seeds, peanut or almond butter or tahini or other nut or seed paste (no added salt)
Milk, yoghurt, cheese and alternatives A standard serve is 500–600kJ	- 1 cup (250ml) fresh, UHT long life, reconstituted powdered milk or buttermilk - ½ cup (120ml) evaporated milk - 2 slices (40g) or 4×3×2cm cube (40g) of hard cheese such as cheddar - ½ cup (120g) ricotta cheese - ¾ cup (200g) yoghurt - 1 cup (250ml) soy, rice or other cereal drink with at least 100mg of calcium per 100ml

The number of recommended serves per age group by sex is presented in the table below. There is a bit of maths involved here to calculate the amount of each food group that is appropriate for your child, allowing for their age and gender. Please set aside time to become familiar with standard serves and healthy portion sizes for you, your child and your family.

Recommended serve sizes		2–3 years	4–8 years	9–11 years	12–13 years	14–18 years
Vegetables & legumes/beans	Boys	2.5	4.5	5	5.5	5.5
	Girls	2.5	4.5	5	5	5
Fruit	Boys	1	1.5	2	2	2
	Girls	1	1.5	2	2	2
Grain (cereal) foods, mostly wholegrain	Boys	4	4	5	6	7
	Girls	4	4	5	6	7
Lean meats and poultry, fish, eggs, tofu, nuts, seeds	Boys	1	1.5	2.5	2.5	2.5
	Girls	1	1.5	2.5	2.5	2.5
Milk, yoghurt, cheese and alternatives	Boys	1.5	2	2.5	3.5	3.5
	Girls	1.5	2	2.5	3.5	3.5

So, for example, the recommended amounts for a five-year-old girl would be:

Food group	Standard size serve multiplied by number of serves	Example of food portion size
Vegetables & legumes/beans	75g or × 4.5 serves	- 1.5 cups green leafy or raw salad vegetables - ½ cup sweet corn - ½ medium potato or other starchy vegetables (sweet potato, taro or cassava) - 1 medium tomato
Fruit	150g × 1.5 serves	- 1 medium apple - 1 apricot
Grain (cereal) foods, mostly wholegrain	500kJ × 4 serves	- 1 slice of bread - ½ cup (125g) cooked porridge - 3 (35g) crispbreads - 1 small English muffin or scone
Lean meats and poultry, fish, eggs, tofu, nuts, seeds	500–600kJ × 1.5 serves	- 100g cooked fish fillet - 1 egg
Milk, yoghurt, cheese and alternatives	500–600kJ × 2 serves	- 1 cup of full-cream milk - ¾ cup (200g) yoghurt

Keep the guide somewhere visible, like on the fridge, that way you won't be guessing when you're preparing meals.

To encourage an increased vegetable intake as per recommended serves, a simple and fun activity for the whole family is starting a basic veggie patch in the backyard or on the sunny balcony. Even a couple of tomato plants in pots on the balcony is a good start. Getting your child involved in the planting may encourage them to be more interested in eating the produce once it's served up on the plate. See www.communitygarden.org.au.

Understanding the glycaemic index

The glycaemic index (GI) was developed by an Australian nutrition researcher Professor Jenny Brandt-Miller at the University of Sydney. In her research, she discovered different foods have different capacities for raising a person's blood sugar. The rate and extent of this rise in blood sugar determines the glycaemic index. Carbohydrates with a low GI value (55 or less) are more slowly digested, absorbed and metabolised, and cause a lower and slower rise in blood glucose and, therefore usually, insulin levels.

What about glycaemic load?

Your blood-glucose levels rise and fall when you eat a meal containing carbohydrates. How high it rises, and how long it stays high, depends on the quality of the carbohydrates (the GI) as well as the quantity of food consumed. Glycaemic load (or GL) combines both the quantity and quality of carbohydrates. It is also the best way to compare blood-glucose values of different types and amounts of foods. The glycaemic load of a food also accounts for the amount of food and associated fibre in the food that is typically eaten as a snack or during a main meal.

Most people don't realise that insulin is the most powerful hormone in the body for driving the development of more fat cells. Reversing these high insulin levels through a changed range of healthy wholefoods containing fibre, vitamins minerals and resistant starches is just another piece of the puzzle for breaking the cycle of obesity.

There is a vast resource of information at the Glycaemic Index Foundation. You can check their website here: www.gisymbol.com

Use their Swap It Tool to swap from higher to lower GI foods: www.gisymbol.com/swap-it

An important note: it is key that you integrate foods with a lower glycaemic index and load into your whole family's diet to reverse insulin resistance or hopefully avoid it developing in the first place. This basically means high-fibre, lower-carbohydrate-containing vegetables such as cauliflower, broccoli, green beans, zucchini, avocado, celery, cabbage and Brussels sprouts – imagine that! As a complication arising from obesity, and now affecting an alarming number of children and teens, type 2 diabetes is completely avoidable. The diet and lifestyle you choose for your child has a direct impact on this outcome.

Let's look at nourishing wholefoods

If you've been out of the loop of preparing wholefoods for your family, now is the ideal time to get back on that bandwagon. It's concerning that many children cannot identify different fruits and vegetables. Jamie Oliver's 'Learn your fruit and veg' program for kids is one great program trying to reverse this: jamiesministryoffood.com.au/our-purpose/jamie-olivers-learn-your-fruit-and-veg. Equally, many parents are unfamiliar with what wholefoods really are. When it's explained to them, it's a real revelation.

Wholefoods are unprocessed foods and include:
- Vegetables
- Fruits
- Wholegrains
- Proteins
- Healthy fats

Working down the list, you should aim to consume wholefoods in that order of magnitude, i.e. first vegetables, then fruits, followed by wholegrains, proteins and fats. You can refer to this list as a guide along with the healthy portion sizes in the table presented on pages 106–109. Now let's explore these whole foods in more detail, especially based on the health benefits of such foods within a Mediterranean diet.[13]

Fruits and vegetables

If you work to the principles of one (for young children) to two (for adolescents and adults) pieces of fruit and up to five different vegetables each day, you're making a great start to including nourishing wholefoods in your diet. We need both fruit and vegetables, and we need them every day.

When I see families in my clinic, I talk to them about creating a rainbow on their plate with the foods they eat. In other words, including foods that have a variety of colours, shapes and textures. Typically, when I first see patients, they are only eating food that is white or brown coloured. I don't have anything against these colours, per se; however, foods coloured this way will impact your child negatively. Brown and white coloured foods (think burgers, chips, cakes and biscuits) will raise blood sugar levels and insulin more quickly and spark the insatiable hunger cycle I described above.

Wholegrains

Most families I see consume grains as white bread, white rice, and processed biscuits, crackers, cereals and cakes. These products are highly refined. When I talk about wholegrains, what I mean is grains that are not refined. You may not be familiar with these, but they include grains such as brown rice, barley, quinoa, polenta and buckwheat. A visit to the wholefoods section of your supermarket or health-food store is a great place to start on the journey to introducing new grains into your family's food regimen.

I recommend to patients to apply the **Just One Thing** rule when integrating new grains. Start with one new grain and experiment with it. Try it in recipes and get confident with how to use it best. Do your research. There is so much information available about healthy wholefoods. Once you've become confident with cooking one new item and your family is enjoying it, introduce another.

Carbohydrates: the healthy versus the unhealthy
So how much carbohydrates should your child and you eat?

Healthy carbohydrates in the form of fresh fruit, vegetables and legumes contain important health-promoting vitamins, minerals and fibre that we all need. The recommended amount of carbohydrate as a macronutrient is between 40 and 60 percent of your total daily calories.[14] Try not to load more than a quarter of your plate with carbs during the day, as when you have, say, a breakfast cereal and a slice of toast or for lunch a sandwich (two pieces of bread for example) you will quickly reach your healthy quota. To keep it simple one should know that one piece of bread or an apple is already 15g. There has been a lot of debate about the benefit of a low carbohydrate diet being an effective weight-loss in adults and perhaps in adolescents.[15, 16] Furthermore it appears in older adults at least, that simply supplementing a Mediterranean-based diet with extra-virgin olive oil or nuts is effective in the prevention of heart attacks and strokes.[17]

Unrefined and unprocessed carbohydrates are an important part of any healthy balanced nutritious diet. However, the reality is that for the children and families I see, carbohydrates are a major driver of their obesity. That is, they consume an excess of refined processed carbohydrates in the form of white bread, white rice, pasta, and snack food like potato and fried chips, and sweet and salty biscuits.

See the resources section at the end of this stage for further resources on low-carb diets.

Eat protein in lean meats and other non-meat sources

The importance of protein has been well established for its ability to maintain good health and support normal growth and development in children and adolescents. The other important role it plays in your family's nutrition is its ability to promote a feeling of fullness or satiety (feeling satisfied after a meal).

Diets lacking adequate amounts of protein lead to hunger and increased total energy intake via overeating of processed foods containing unhealthy carbohydrates and fats (the so-called protein leverage hypothesis of Professors Evan Simpson and David Raubenheimer at The University of Sydney).[18] Lean meats include: lean red meats (beef, lamb and veal), white meats (pork, chicken and turkey) and fish. Understanding that meat is a more expensive inclusion in family meals, you may need to get creative. Some of the cheapest cuts of meat are the tastiest, but simply require longer cooking times. Just ask your local butcher! (If you have one still in your neighbourhood!)

Or see these guides:
www.australianbeef.com.au/know-your-meat/butchers-guide-to-popular-beef-cuts
www.australianlamb.com.au/know-your-meat/lamb-cuts-chart
www.porkstar.com.au/secret-recipe-booklets
www.goodfish.org.au/resources/

For non-meat-based sources of protein, think eggs, tofu, nuts, legumes (chickpeas, lentils) and beans. Check out these resources:
www.veganaustralia.org.au
www.nutritionaustralia.org/national/frequently-asked-questions/vegetarian-diets

Again, if you're unfamiliar with these foods, apply the **Just One Thing** rule. Experiment and build your confidence as you build these new ingredients into your family's food regimen.

Healthy fats

There is an ongoing reappraisal of the role of healthy fats in health and disease, and this book doesn't allow for a full exploration of this contentious discussion; however, I do offer some thoughts here.

Back when your great-grandmother prepared real food, she cooked with real healthy fats like real butter, full-fat milk and cream, and animal fats (such as lard and dripping). During the seventies, under the influence of legitimate concerns about the increased prevalence of heart disease, fats in our diet became enemy number one.

Sadly, this led to the artificial-food industry promoting processed, so-called low-fat foods. The problem was, and remains, the taste of these foods was enhanced by the addition of highly refined sugars. It was necessary to do this because when removing fats from food much of the flavour and the properties that cause you to feel full when you eat it are also stripped away. The net effect is people have been living under the illusion they are eating more healthily because they're eating low fat, when in fact their high sugar intake is causing them to become sick and perpetuate the cycle of obesity. The irony is this is what they were trying to avoid in the first place. Welcome to the world of food marketing!

While it seems paradoxical to most families I see in my clinic, incorporating the right amount healthy fats into the family's food is a critical step to break the cycle of obesity. Is this an open invitation to consume lots of fats? No, it isn't. But it's important to recognise healthy fats are essential in every diet and like every other element, must be consumed in the appropriate balance. We should also make the distinction between healthy fats and unhealthy fats. Without getting too technical, healthy fats are:

- Polyunsaturated fats such as fish oil, flaxseed oil, safflower and sunflower seed oil
- Monounsaturated fats, including olive oil, canola oil, most nuts.

The good news is these oils are readily available in supermarkets. As demand for healthy fats has grown, especially within a Mediterranean diet, has grown (see www.mediterraneanbook.com), the price of these oils has made them more financially accessible for every budget. Be sure to add these to your shopping list. You can use the table of nuts and seeds containing healthy fats as a guide for helping you decide which are the healthiest for you.[19]

Food (28g serving)	Calories	Total fat (g)	Food (28g serving)	Calories	Total fat (g)
Almonds	169	15	Olives, ripe, canned	32	3
Avocado	50	4.5	Peanuts	164	14
Brazil nuts	185	19	Pecans	199	21
Cashews	155	12	Pine nuts	190	19
Chia seeds	137	9	Pistachios	157	13
Flax seeds	150	12	Pumpkin seeds	153	13
Hazelnuts	181	18	Sesame seeds	160	14
Hemp seeds	160	12	Sunflower seeds	163	14
Macadamia nuts	203	22	Walnuts	185	18

Water

No healthy food discussion would be complete without mention of the importance of drinking water. It's almost so obvious we can overlook it for optimal health and wellbeing. Water has many functions in our body: it aids digestion, prevents constipation, normalises blood pressure and stabilises the heartbeat.[20]

While our need for water has not changed, its consumption has been superseded by consumption of sugar-sweetened beverages, including all soft drinks, cordials, fruit juice, fizzy drinks and so-called sports drinks, sales of which have grown in recent decades. What we don't realise is that many of us are dehydrated and don't know it, and these sugary drinks are contributing to that state.

Just remember simply cutting out one can of soft drink (which contains about 12 teaspoons of sugar) a day and replacing it with fresh water can help the average person (child or adult) not gain about 3kg in the next year! You might argue that the zero sugar or diet options are better than the full-sugar-containing soft drinks, but good evidence suggests such 'diet' soft drinks increase your appetite and may still predispose you to increased weight gain and diabetes risk.

As you work towards breaking the cycle of obesity in your family, stick to water as the main liquid refreshment. You will find, within a very short space of time, your taste will evolve to this far healthier alternative. You will also notice the savings you'll make when you shop (money you can spend on healthier alternatives), as well as the fewer fights about what to drink and the change in the way you feel from the reduced sugar intake.

Your new healthy eating plan

Now that you've absorbed the information in this stage, you can approach your shopping list and menu plan with an intention of buying nourishing wholefoods to use in home-cooked meals.

Initially, you may struggle to find replacements for the familiar foods you typically cook and eat. Fortunately, there is a way around that block. FoodSwitch is a website and app that empowers consumers to find healthy alternatives to the less nutritious items they've been consuming. The website is a treasure trove of resources, providing easy-to-understand information about packaged foods products, as well as similar foods that are healthier choices. FoodSwitch uses a traffic light labelling system making it possible to identify the suitability of a food for your family.

What does breastfeeding have to do with breaking the cycle of obesity?

It might seem strange to mention breastfeeding in a book about breaking the cycle of obesity but many mums who see me in the clinic often have more than one child and are contemplating having more. If this is you, then breastfeeding is where you can start to learn about the way food nourishes your child.

Breastfeeding is a wonderful opportunity for a mother and infant to bond. Mothers can learn vital clues about their child's appetite through the routine of breastfeeding. Notwithstanding the physical challenges some mums may have, if it's at all possible, I recommend breastfeeding for at least the first six months of your child's life. Obviously, if you can breastfeed longer and you're continuing to enjoy the experience of closeness and nurturing it brings to your relationship with your infant, I would encourage you to continue for longer.

If you are the mother of an infant (i.e. your child is three years or younger), it is important to be aware that during this critical time of your child's growth and development, they are acquiring lifelong skills and behaviours, which will influence their risk of obesity and chronic diseases such as diabetes. During this time children learn to recognise when they have eaten enough to be satisfied. They also adopt food preferences that are either healthy or unhealthy. Your critical role as a mother in this process cannot be overstated.

In my clinic, I see so many mothers of infants who have been unable to recognise when their child has eaten enough to be satisfied. Not an easy thing to learn, it requires that the mother 'mind read' the cues from the child before the child can articulate these themselves.

Establishing healthy eating early, including breastfeeding, will help arrest the cycle of obesity. While breastfeeding per se may not necessarily prevent your individual child becoming overweight or obese, in the presence of many other drivers of weight gain during childhood, its many other benefits are clear. If you're the mother of an infant, consider reading *Born to Eat* by Leslie Schilling and Wendy Jo Peterson.

I appreciate a mountain of information has been shared in this stage. In fact, it would be easy to write a whole book just on this topic alone, but remember you are working to principles and developing your own wisdom about food. Be patient because it will take time.

Resources

Make sure you also get across to the Ride to Life website and access all the online resources that are available there.

While I am not enamoured necessarily with the name of the website www.dietdoctor.com,[21] it has scientifically validated information on low-carbohydrate dietary approaches. The site also has great low-carbohydrate recipes and colourful visual guides that may be useful to some of you. As I mentioned earlier, aim to keep it simple and, if you wish to pursue the approaches suggested by www.dietdoctor.com, always seek medical and nutritional advice first before starting.

Check out these great healthy cooking videos on YouTube and online from Australia and overseas from Kaiser Permanente USA: www.youtube.com/watch?v=Oh10CJshlis&list=

We Can! is an excellent American general healthy lifestyle website: www.nhlbi.nih.gov/health/educational/wecan/index.htm

Find this excellent simple recipe book from the National Institute of Health: healthyeating.nhlbi.nih.gov/pdfs/Dinners_Cookbook_508-compliant.pdf

Jamie Oliver is great on YouTube for quick but nutritious meals: www.youtube.com/user/JamieOliver. Look out for his one-minute cooking tips!

Edible Education by American Ann Butler is about educating children to cook healthy real food: edibleedu.com

Check out our own national treasure Stephanie Alexander's the kitchen garden program: www.kitchengardenfoundation.org.au

Donna Hay's cooking show *Basics to Brilliance Kids* is marvelous: www.sbs.com.au/food/article/2019/01/10/donna-hay-basics-brilliance-kids-episode-guide-and-recipes, www.sbs.com.au/food/program/donna-hay-basics-brilliance-kids

Simply Recipes (USA) is another good resource: www.simplyrecipes.com/recipes/type/quick

Good and Cheap: Eat well on $4 a day by Leanne Brown. What an amazingly inspiring project and New York lady, with great affordable recipes for those on a limited budget, but shouldn't that be all of us? (books.leannebrown.com/good-and-cheap.pdf)

For more health and nutrition information and resources:

The New South Wales Healthy Kids website: www.healthykids.nsw.gov.au/ has some of the best health information to help families eat healthily and stay active. Under the 'Campaigns and Programs' link you will find many of the NSW Health initiatives to promote healthy weight and prevent overweight and obesity in families.

The Heart Foundation has just released their latest recommendation for healthy eating, with lots of great and advice and recipes: www.heartfoundation.org.au/healthy-eating/food-and-nutrition

Diabetes NSW: www.diabetesnsw.com.au/about-diabetes

Diabetes Australia: www.diabetesaustralia.com.au

Nutrition Council of Australia recipes: www.nutritioncouncilaustralia.com.au/recipes

Nutrition Australia: www.nutritionaustralia.org

Notes

Notes

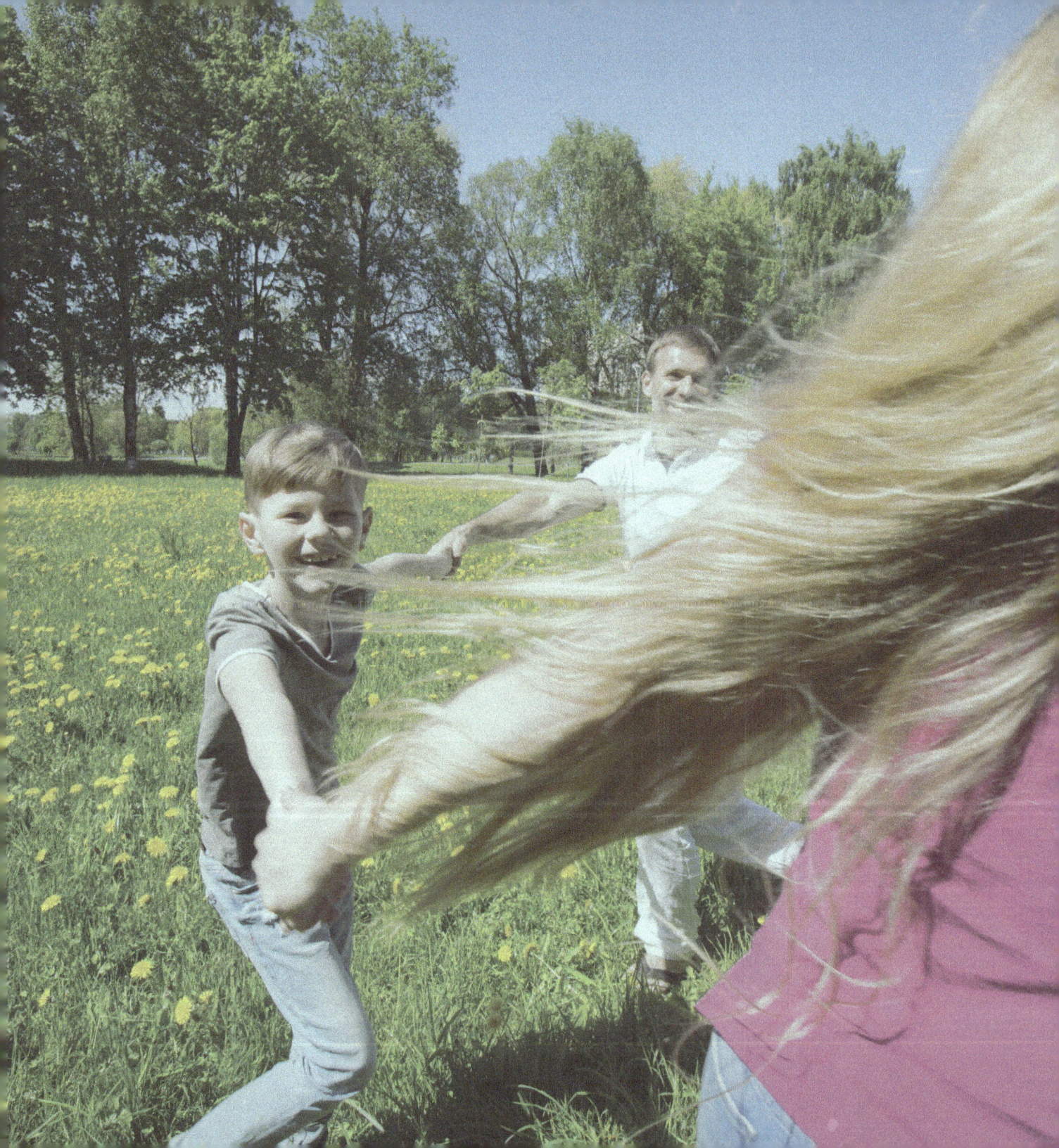

Stage 6

Get moving! Learning to love exercise and move your body consciously!

> *Those who do not find time for exercise will have to find time for illness*
>
> Proverb

> *Action is movement with intelligence. The world is filled with movement. What the world needs is more conscious movement, more action.*
>
> Sri B.K.S Iyengar, Yogi and Founder of Iyengar School of Yoga

No discussion about overcoming obesity would be complete without mentioning the requirement for physical activity or simply moving more rather than sitting – that is, reducing sedentary behaviours at work and home, usually in front of a screen of some sort. That's why, along with many others shared in this book, I'm happy to include yet another tried and true statement. Evidence of the multiple benefits of regular physical activity is well documented.

In this stage, which focuses on getting moving, we will:

- ■ Highlight the mental and physical health benefits of regular physical activity.
- ■ Explain the damaging effects caused by an excessively sedentary lifestyle.
- ■ Explore the importance of the natural world in promoting health and wellbeing.

Why is moving important?

Research has shown healthy physical activity reduces the risk of chronic diseases such as type 2 diabetes, heart disease, osteoporosis and mental illness. It also enhances body balance and prevents falls and dementia. While the jury is still out as to whether high-intensity physical activity relative to low-intensity physical activity is better in the promotion of health, particularly in relation to type 2 diabetes prevention, there is no question that moving in any way is better than not moving at all. Regardless of the type of physical activity undertaken, it is apparent all forms of physical activity, in adequate amounts performed at the right intensity level, provide significant health benefits.

Not convinced? Well, it seems there are many with a similar mindset who also don't like exercise.

The reality is, in our modern society, with the prevalence of technology and the less physical nature of work for most people, the majority of the population do not do enough physical activity. This is particularly striking in childhood and adolescence as we now find there are many children and teenagers who do no exercise at all, spending far too much time being sedentary (usually on technology of some form).

Remember when your child first learnt to crawl and then walk? There was excitement when they took their first steps. This desire for movement in humans is natural and instinctive. It is a tragedy in our modern society that this natural instinct has been suppressed by changes in lifestyle, diet and values. The instinct to move, which allows the child to develop a love of physical activity, occurs during the critical first years of life, making it an imperative for parents to recognise this and encourage physical play from birth, and preferably outdoors surrounded by the wonders of the natural world.

Lack of exercise or sedentariness (sitting around and not moving, basically) is now recognised as an independent risk factor for many chronic diseases including heart disease, diabetes, mental illness (depression and anxiety) and even cancer, and associated with increased mortality and reduced life expectancy.[22]

This sounds shocking but it's not surprising to me as every day in my clinic I see what excessive screen time in children, especially adolescents, and their parents does to their levels of physical and mental fitness!

The World Health Organization has recognised physical inactivity as such a threat to risk for chronic diseases and global health that it has developed a global strategy for getting more of us moving and active over the next ten years: www.who.int/ncds/prevention/physical-activity/gappa/

Screen time

We all enjoy watching a bit of TV or the odd movie – I personally love the old Charlie Chaplin silent movies! Keeping in touch with friends via Facebook and Skype can be rewarding and fun, but also time-consuming and addictive. Not all screen time is bad for kids by any means, especially if you are engaged with them at the time. Playing computer games can promote problem-solving skills and might give them new ideas for traditional play. But the flipside of screen time is the lost opportunity for physical activity out in the sun or rain in a natural place, and thus the potential for disconnection from the real world.

	PARENT 1		PARENT 2		CHILD 1		CHILD 2		CHILD 3	
	Type	Duration (hours)	Type	Duration (hours)	Type	Duration (hours)	Type	Duration (hours)	Type	Duration (hours)
Monday										
Tuesday										
Wednesday										
Thursday										
Friday										
Saturday AM										
Saturday PM										
Sunday AM										
Sunday PM										

Complete the table above to review how much time you and your family are spending in front of a TV, computer, phone, or on social media and other technologies.

At the end of a long day you might be looking forward to curling up on the couch with your favourite TV show while flicking through Instagram, but consider the frequency and overall time spent being sedentary.

The latest guidelines from the American Academy of Pediatrics (AAP) suggest the following:

- Children under 18 months should avoid screen time.
- Children aged 18 months to two years can watch or use high-quality programs or apps if adults watch or play with them to help them understand what they're seeing.
- Children aged two to five years should have no more than one hour a day of screen time with adults watching or playing with them.
- Children aged six years and older should have consistent limits on the time they spend on electronic media and the types of media they use.

I know this is really difficult for some parents to switch off the internet connection (I found it really hard myself), but I am aghast when I see a young parent pushing their infant child around in the pram in the street, with the parent looking at his or her iPhone and half their time the child is also looking at an iPad or some device! Double disconnection! This is a lost opportunity for you and your child to talk, make funny noises and laugh together!

Please don't waste the valuable time you have with your children; they grow up very fast and before you know they have left you and you wonder, what did I do to deserve their inattention?

Consider establishing some reasonable limits around screen time. For example, after school no TV before 5pm. Having some no TV days during the week and weekend. You can negotiate this with your children (and your partner!) as they will be hesitant and resistant at first, but link it to some healthy rewards and goals at the end of month or quarter – that is, they get to earn some frequent-flyer healthy points towards some family adventure, holiday as a family, or a day outing to a theme park, beach or national park! Just use your imagination, and it does not have to be a five-star expensive holiday to Disneyland! Just spending time together as a family is so valuable.

It's also important to note that it is not your job to entertain your child every second of the day. Ellyn Satter highlights the importance of children being responsible for dealing with their own boredom in the absence of technology/screen solution. Boredom creates imagination but as a parent you have to provide some simple resources for your child's imagination to blossom. You can provide age-appropriate resources such as coloured pencils and drawing books (mindful colouring books or puzzles can be great fun), paint, playdough, dress ups or toys that encourage open-ended play. Or for older kids, get them to the local park for some ball games or a bike ride. They might be independent enough that you can build trust with them to let them go with friends or a sibling. This is something you as a parent need to explore.

Positive impacts of exercise

In the same way the impact of these sedentary behaviours are felt long after they're over, the benefits of physical activity, can be enjoyed well past the time the activity is undertaken. Exercise is well recognised for its ability to up-regulate chemicals in the brain which promote feelings of wellbeing and positivity. And when I say exercise, I mean bodily physical activity involving movement. This can range from simple walking, stretching or more vigorous activities such as cycling, running and various traditional sports to other less conventional forms of exercise. Singing, for example, is a powerful emotional and spiritual activity, especially when singing in a group. It's also very good for the body as it positively impacts on your breathing and diaphragm.

Check out Creativity Australia (www.creativityaustralia.org.au) where the benefits of choir singing are explained. Dr K had the pleasure of meeting Tanya de Jong, AM, the inspiring founder.

As important to a person's wellbeing are the mental health promoting effects of physical activity. In my own experience, riding my bicycle regularly has had enormous beneficial impact on my mental health. In fact, apart from keeping me fit, I would say for me, riding my bike is the best antidepressant on the market. There is ample science to back up the mental/emotional benefits of physical activity and you can read more about this if you choose. You don't really need to understand the science. Just know, for you and your family to break the cycle of obesity, daily physical activity is an essential ingredient in recovery and enjoying life and all that it has to offer with family and friends.

Getting started

Enjoying the benefits of exercise may not occur on your first attempt at becoming more active, but it will happen if you're consistent. It's a bit like brushing your teeth. If you only did it once a week for a couple of minutes, you couldn't really expect to have good oral health. But if you brush your teeth for two minutes twice a day, every day, you will definitely notice a difference in your oral and general health because the two are interlinked.

Like anything, where new patterns of behaviour are being established, it takes time to integrate and see the results manifest on the physical plane. But rest assured regular daily exercise (even 15 minutes to start off with, as you build up to at least 60 minutes a day for your child) of being more active will lead to improvements in fitness and their enjoyment within a very short time! Futhermore, once you have the experience of a changing physical body that can cope better with more physical demands it will become easier to adhere to a regular physical activity routine. Those initial sore muscles and joints will remind you that you need to be more active and will soon turn into feelings of strength and power and an urge to move more, faster and longer! You just have to accept that there will be some pain and that this pain may be good for you! With one more day of moving, you and your child will build confidence and a greater, deeper well of energy, and you will start enjoying the moving feelings! It always works for Dr Koala.

> Remember, physical activity on its own may not necessarily help you lose weight; however, it does prevent weight gain and is an essential part of a healthy body, mind and life.

Before you launch into an exercise program, it pays to consider why you haven't been exercising prior to this point. Many people suffering from obesity – parents and children alike – have negative associations with exercise and resist doing it at all costs. If you're to integrate physical activity into your family's life, we need to explore the origins of this resistance.

What if you hate exercise?

Without wanting to sound like a taskmaster, if you hate exercise and want to break the cycle of obesity in your family you will have to find a way to work through this resistance and overcome it. If this sounds like a harsh reality, it's because it is. Remember, in this book we're dealing with honesty and the truth is you and your family will need to get moving.

Tick whichever of these apply to you as reasons for holding you back from being active:

☐ Low self-esteem and fear of being teased/bullied – 'Look at that fat kid trying to exercise! Doesn't he look funny sweating and puffing away.'

☐ Pain in the body, perhaps legs and back, from exercise. This is normal, but for many very obese kids it can be a real deterrent.

☐ Fear of sweating excessively, leading you to perceive this as body odour problems which again links to fear of being teased. This fear is particularly heightened in girls.

☐ Concerns about not being able to keep up with those annoying 'skinny kids' – especially in competition sports and a feeling of being overlooked by the coaches. This can build up to feelings of 'failure' and low self-esteem.

☐ Body image – do you have rolls of fat on your tummy which embarrass you? In boys pendulous breasts can be a big barrier to swimming in summer. Girls with a large waist may struggle to find appropriate beachwear that feels becoming.

If you hate exercise, take some time to reflect on why that is. For example, I have many parents who tell me that as a teenager, they weren't confident sportspeople, so they gave up doing anything at all. The reality is you're no longer a teenager and therefore no longer subject to peer bullying or criticism for a lack of sporting or physical prowess. Besides, who said you needed to be a superstar at a sport? You don't need to be amazing at sport to enjoy kicking a ball around the park with your children, or playing on the see-saw, or going for a simple walk together as a family! Enjoy moving together as best you can. The more regularly you build this into your weekly timetable the more you will enjoy it.

Use your influence wisely

Know that as the parent, you have immense power to influence your child's perception of anything, including physical activity. If you project a negative perception of it, guess what? They will take it on board too. And it's not enough to tell them to be more physical, particularly when you aren't a physically active role model yourself. As the parent, it is your responsibility to lead the child and adolescent towards a healthier, more active life. I am not saying it is easy, but I encourage you to have the necessary courage to take steps forward.

I find many families rely upon the father to engage the children in physical activity, while the mother focuses on other aspects of running the family. The downside of this is when the father is physically inactive himself and one or both parents are obese because this entrenches a sedentary inactive family lifestyle for everyone. It is very difficult to overcome this barrier to a family becoming active. In my clinical experience, it only occurs to the parents that they might need to change this approach after the experience of a major health crisis. Usually this presents as an early heart attack or the diagnosis of diabetes in one of the parents (usually the father). I don't know about you, but I'd prefer to get moving now rather than wait for the heart attack to occur first!

Why doesn't your child do physical activity?

Now that you have assessed why you as a parent aren't physically active, consider the situation from your child's perspective. Aside from your influence, can you pinpoint what else might be holding them back? Think about emotional factors, but also scheduling and practical considerations.

- Does your child feel self-conscious about participating in a team sport because they feel they 'lack' sporting abilities and may be embarrassed to let the team down?
- Do they feel isolated due to their obesity and are disinclined to get involved in team sports? Were they bullied at some time during a PE class at school or at a swimming lesson? Were they picked on or humiliated by a sports coach or teacher or another student?
- Do they spend a lot of time indoors studying or using technology?
- Do they have a lot of indoor commitments like music lessons or other academic pursuits which limit their time?
- Is there a lack of outdoor play area and equipment (trampoline, bouncy ball, cricket bat or tennis racquet) around your home?
- Are there parks or appropriate outdoor play areas near your home where they can spend time or is your neighbourhood not suitable for outdoor activity for some reason?
- Is your child always driven to school and other activities, rather than walking or catching public transport (if old and responsible enough)?
- Have you nurtured that responsibility or found it difficult to let go as your child has grown older?

There was nothing more fun (in my own personal experience as a father) than when I was taking my kids to the park or beach, and playing games and rolling in the grass with them. It is a wonderful bonding experience and kids love it if you can spend one-on-one time with them after school and on weekends doing 'crazy', fun stuff together with a laugh and a huff and puff!

Overcoming resistance and barriers

If you've done the exercise above you will have identified your resistance to physical activity as well as some barriers that your child might be facing too. While I appreciate it may be uncomfortable getting out there and being seen if you're not completely comfortable in your skin yet, the bottom line is this: we're talking about saving people's lives here – yours and your child's. What's more, there are other people doing it, taking responsibility for their health and that of their family, and moving.

In order to overcome your mental barrier, revisit your why! Your why will motivate you to let go of your resistance and hold on to your motivation for making changes in your life. To help your child feel more motivated, talk to them about what kind of activity they might find enjoyable. No one is looking to make your child feel vulnerable or embarrassed. The first activity might be as simple as walking the dog, walking part of the way to school with them, or going to the local park to kick a ball.

Assessment of what you do now

The following provides an overview of the guidelines for various exercise types and the corresponding intensity levels.[23]

- The intensity level of an activity relates to how hard the body works during that activity.
- Activity levels are referred to as light, moderate or vigorous.
- Metabolic equivalent is the term used to express the intensity of physical activities.

Moderate intensity	Vigorous intensity
Requires a moderate amount of effort and noticeably accelerates the heart rate	Requires a large amount of effort and causes rapid breathing and a substantial increase in heart rate
Examples of moderate-intensity exercise: • Brisk walking • Dancing • Gardening • Housework or domestic chores • Active involvement in games and sports with children/walking pets • General building tasks (e.g. roofing, painting) • Carrying/moving moderate loads (←20kg)	Examples of vigorous-intensity exercise: • Running • Walking briskly up a hill • Cycling up a hill • Aerobics • Fast swimming • Competitive sports and games (e.g. traditional games, football, volleyball, hockey, basketball) • Heavy shovelling or digging ditches • Carrying/moving heavy loads (→20kgs)

Complete the table below and identify who does what in terms of physical activity in your family. What physical activities does each member of the family do during the week and weekend? What type, duration and intensity (low, moderate, vigorous)?

	PARENT 1		PARENT 2		CHILD 1		CHILD 2		CHILD 3	
	Type/Intensity	Duration (hours)	Type/Intensity	Duration (hours)	Type/Intensity	Duration (hours)	Type/Intensity	Duration (hours)	Type/Intensity	Duration (hours)
Monday										
Tuesday										
Wednesday										
Thursday										
Friday										
Saturday AM										
Saturday PM										
Sunday AM										
Sunday PM										

Let's get physical

Just as we created the right space for mindful meals, you need to create the right conditions for integrating regular physical activity into your life. Fortunately, physical activity comes in many forms. There are myriad options and, like we did with our food principles, it's necessary for you to tune into your inner wisdom about what works for you and your child. This will require patience and persistence as you experiment to find what works best. Remember that not all children are naturally 'sporty' and there's nothing wrong with that. We're not trying to force a child who doesn't feel comfortable or confident to join a swimming team or to do something that will make them feel anxious or exposed. What we're trying to do is encourage some – *any* – form of physical activity that gets them moving. As with other aspects of your health journey, it's time to bring some creativity to the equation, especially if your family's habit is not to exercise.

When families come to see me in the clinic, one of the exercises I do with them is ask if they know the locations of their local parks or active outdoor areas. It continually surprises me how few families know the location of their closest park or active outdoor area. Nor are they aware of the local youth clubs, like Scouts, YMCA or PCYC, or their local Park Run, all of which offer relatively inexpensive healthy activities. Essential to reclaiming your life and breaking the cycle of obesity in your family is the inclusion of physical activity done together as part of daily and weekly routines.

Choosing an activity

There are many activity options; however, some underlying principles should be kept in mind when making your selection:

- **Your choice of exercise should be enjoyable.** It may take time to reach a point where it becomes easily enjoyable and fun, but you will get there if you persist.
- **Preferably choose activities that can be done outside in a natural environment.** This has the additional beneficial effects of providing a connection to nature's healing properties, including vitamin D from the sun and the calming power of listening, seeing, touching and smelling the wonder of the natural world. One of my favourite authors is Richard Louv, author of *Vitamin N* – highly recommended for nature therapy!
- **Find activities you can do with an encouraging friend or a community group.** It is always easier to take the first step to an active life if you have someone to share it with. You will find that making a commitment to a time, place and activity will keep you both

honest. I know that if my riding buddy George and I agree to meet at 6.30am, even if it's cold and dark and I'm tired and feel like staying in bed for another half an hour, my commitment to meet George gets me out of bed and on my bike every time. I don't want to let him down, and once I'm out there I am always so glad I stuck to my commitment. You will have the same experience when you set up a similar arrangement with your active partner.

- **Be consistent with your activity.** To break the cycle of obesity, consistent physical activity is a must. Once a week won't cut it. (Remember my analogy of only brushing your teeth once?) Working towards being physically active every day is your goal.
To achieve this level of activity, you will need to engage your imagination about the activities you'll attempt, enjoy and persist with. Like anything in life, variety will help to keep you interested and inspired. You may also need to find more than one active buddy to join you. Even a virtual on-line active buddy helps you get motivated. I've tried the cycle and running app Zwift!; it works to get you out of bed, especially on a rainy morning when an indoor cycle trainer or treadmill is dryer and safer!

- **Engage the family.** Breaking the cycle of obesity in your family means *everyone* needs to be active, not just you. Although it might start with just you, find ways to facilitate the involvement of each family member, taking into account their age and stage of development and readiness to participate. If you have a partner, it may require having a hard conversation about 'one in, all in'. If this is difficult, remember your '**Why**' and keep moving. It will be worth it. You may need to get support for navigating this conversation and the changes that ensue.

- **Have zero tolerance for excuses.** Apart from emergency situations and extreme circumstances beyond your control, do not go down the road of excuses for getting out of your exercise regimen. It is highly likely this will take all your resolve and it's where your '**Why**', your active buddies and your commitment to Ride to Life will keep you going.

What kind of activity might work for you and your family?

Here are a few ideas to get you going. Remember, you don't need to run a marathon in week one. Remember the **Just One Thing** rule. Start with something small and slowly integrate it into your routine.

- A walk to the shops. Out of milk? Walk 10–15 minutes to the local milk bar and enjoy the fresh air, rather than drive the car, so also helping reduce global warming!
- A trip to the local park. If possible walk or scooter or ride your bikes with your child to the park. You might take a kite, football, frisbee or your dear dog who may also have put on too much weight recently.
- Basic ball sports with Dad and Mum. Grab a footy or soccer or tennis ball and kick and throw it around the backyard or local park for a 30 minute active session before or after dinner (in summer time when cooler later in the day). Doesn't matter if you are not Adam Goodes, Diego Maradona or Roger Federer, you're just trying to have a bit of fun together and you *will* improve with practice.

Family Story

Happy smiling active Polly

Polly was a single child of two caring, lovely parents. She gained weight very quickly in primary school so she was already 70kg by 10 years old. Her mother was also obese, worked full-time and struggled with eating healthily. Although Polly loved soccer (her father was the coach), large intakes of processed packaged foods and sweets, and large portion sizes contributed to her weight gain and the development of obesity in early childhood.

Through reduced consumption of packaged foods, fewer takeaway dinners and junk food, more water, more daily regular physical activity, walks with family on the weekend, more active transport to school (sometimes walking part of the way to and from school), swimming in summer, and less screen time her weight gain slowed significantly. Her mother also attended clinical psychology and nutrition sessions for herself at our clinic. Overall the whole family moved to a healthier, happier place in their lives and developed a healthier more mindful attitude to food and an enjoyment of being more physically active. What a great outcome for this family.

Don't forget about local kids' organisations such as Scouts, Girl Guides and YMCA. There is also one that is inexpensive and usually running in most neighbourhoods: PCYC. They have great programs such as kids' boxing and martial arts programs. If you are lucky enough to be near the water, you might consider kids' sailing lessons and nippers as part of surf lifesaving.

You can explore nature itself using this great app: www.natureplaywa.org.au/.

One of my patient's Mother put me onto this app and they found it really motivated their children to get outdoors and explore their local natural environment and beyond!

Incidental activity

Incidental activity is the way you move every moment of the day, from the time you get out of bed, get to work, move at work, and get home. For example, think about how many stairs you come across each day. Do you take the stairs or the lift or escalator? When you park at the supermarket, do you park as close as possible to the supermarket entrance or deliberately park further away to give you the opportunity to walk a few extra steps? Can you go for a 10 or 15-minute walk during your lunch break to get outside, and feel the sun and breeze on your face? These are not significant activities, but together they all make for a more active person and will keep you healthy. I tell my patients, if you must take the escalator then stand on the right side and walk up; don't just stand there like most people do. Get moving! Be proud that you're taking another step in the right direction.

A note about incidental exercise: don't make it your total physical activity quotient, but do make it part of your mindset. A good rule of thumb is if there's an opportunity to move then take it.

If you drive your child to school or other activities, consider whether they or you both could walk (or bike ride!) part of the way. Could you add in an outdoor activity pre or post other commitments? For example, if your child has a music class on a Saturday morning, could you find a park close to the lesson venue and spend an hour playing there afterwards? Or while your child is having their music lesson go for a walk or run or bike ride yourself to build up your steps and fitness, breathe in that fresh air and enjoy hopefully some sunshine, rather than sitting in a coffee shop having another – what do they call it – muggocinno!

Remember, even though you're becoming more active, it is still essential you adjust your food and nutrition accordingly. One without the other will not be enough to break the cycle of obesity. Unless you're running marathons every week, you cannot ignore what you feed yourself and your family. That means healthier food, probably smaller portions, less sugar intake, and eating mindfully and enjoyably.

A word of caution: before beginning any exercise regimen, be sure to consult with your regular general practitioner or treating specialist if you have one. At the very least, this will provide a solid reference point as you move towards a healthier you. They can also provide support as you and your family step forward to healthier, happier lives.

Start simple

Like the area of food, with physical activity there is always more information you can find to get you on the road to better health and wellbeing. Rather than spend a huge amount of time doing that, I encourage you to just get moving every day.

Family Story

Omir's story: a common but positive struggle

Omir comes from a Lebanese family. I first saw him in my clinic when he was seven-and-a-half years old.

He had suffered from very poorly controlled asthma for two–three years and had undergone multiple hospital admissions, with many courses of oral prednisone. This had stimulated his appetite, made him gain large amounts of weight and severely restricted his exercise capacity. With improvement in the management of his asthma through preventers (inhaled steroids) he was able to start playing rugby, training twice a week with a game on Saturdays. He was otherwise very sedentary. Although his screen time was generally less than two hours a day, he preferred to sit around.

By age seven years and five months, his weight was 64kg, with a waist circumference of 94cm and body mass index of $35.2 kg/m^2$ in the extreme obesity range and at very high risk of type 2 diabetes and fatty liver disease.

He already had several complications related to his severe obesity, including obstructive sleep apnoea and insulin resistance, with a typical black-coloured rash on his neck and in his armpits called *acanthosis nigricans*. Blood tests revealed he also had high insulin levels consistent with a state of insulin resistance.

Omir was a very fussy eater and basically ate adult-size portions in a fast, mindless manner, finishing his main meals in less than ten minutes. He did not like eating vegetables and had large intake of carbohydrates in the form of pasta. His mother tried her best but struggled to deal with Omir who ate too much and her younger four-year-old son, who was perceived by his mother to be underweight and a fussy eater, who did not eat enough (actually he was in the healthy weight range).

Omir's father worked for a juice company as a manager so was very busy. Mum had stopped soft drinks and juice in the house and switched Omir to water only and encouraged him to eat smaller portions, less carbs and more fresh vegetables with healthy proteins and fibre.

Omir had already been started on a small dose of metformin, a drug used for treatment of type 2 diabetes and insulin resistance.

Over the year he and his mother saw me in my clinic, Omir continued to gain weight until he was 75.5kg as initial changes in reducing portion sizes, pasta and bread intake and encouraging more fresh vegetables in snacks and at dinner time lasted only a month or so.

He also stopped his metformin tablets as he refused to take them.

His lovely mother was very determined though after seeing that he had gained 11kg weight in 10 months and, with encouragement, she tried again to make healthier changes in his nutrition and enrolled in him and his brothers in a local gymnasium for jujitsu, boxing and fitness classes three to four times a week. Over the last few months he lost 0.7kg (which may not seem much, but even no weight gain or a small loss can be a blessing for a boy like Omir).

Omir's mum has been sending me photos of his dinner and gym sessions and, though there are some not-so-good days, overall they are making progress – a trial of steamed broccoli with his chicken was eaten but vomited up after 15 minutes!

Slower mindful eating has been encouraged. Mum has been strong by only giving the whole family healthier choices with 50 percent vegetables and fresh rainbow food, and less carbohydrates served on smaller plates. This is the key to sustainable changes. Omir's dad has been supporting his wife's changes and has been involved in taking him to weekend outdoor physical activities as well. This family and Omir's health journey is going to be a life-long one. His exposure to high-dose steroids in early childhood certainly predisposed him to lasting changes in his metabolism, eating habits and appetite so it will be a struggle, but real food and minimising processed, packaged food and carb intake is essential for this boy's long-term health. His mother has a great deal of determination and has to stay resilient as to why she wants to make these changes for her son and her whole family.

Omir's mum's words on her struggles with Omir and her family

> *It's not easy being a parent; it comes with a big and very important responsibility, especially when it comes to your kids' health. I am a mother of three beautiful boys. One of my boys is underweight and one is overweight.*

It's been really hard and very challenging putting Omir on a diet; he is a very fussy eater and hates vegetables. Coming from a Lebanese background, we love food. Every month, Omir was gaining two to three kilos. I'm heartbroken over my son. I have tried so hard to put him on a diet and I have tried so many ways and so many diets as I'm desperate for him to lose weight.

The hardest day of my life was when I found out Omir had high insulin – that just broke me. I just felt like I had failed: I had failed Omir. Looking into his eyes and looking at him was like my heart getting ripped out of my body. Knowing he is close to having diabetes, I just couldn't handle it. I cried for the whole day and every night I cried myself to sleep. It was honestly so hard to sleep at night because I'd think and think so I'd get up and I'd pray and pray for God to help me and to give me the strength to stand strong next to Omir and help him lose weight.

I made a promise to myself that I won't break down anymore, that I will give him all that I can and will do whatever it takes for Omir to lose weight. I will support him and motivate him for the rest of my life.

It's been a roller-coaster with Omir's diet. There have been a lot of ups and downs. Sometimes I feel scared of giving up hope. I always try to think positive. All I think of is Omir and his weight and how to help him. I sit on the computer and search on different websites for hours; I go to the shops and spend at least two hours in Woolies reading the back of everything before putting it in my trolley.

With Omir, I have been watching on YouTube about overweight kids and how they lose weight and it has really motivated us both. We are both excited at the end result and are working as a team, though there are days tougher than other days, but it's all about being patient. Balancing between my overweight son and my underweight son has been really life-changing for me. It's difficult, but I'm a fighter; even if I fall a few times I manage to get back up and keep going. I have learnt in my life not to rely on anybody but myself. All my time is on my kids. I bought Omir a scale so he can keep track of his weight and it's helped him and motivated him to lose weight step by step. Omir is learning to get on a healthier diet and I'm so proud of him. I will continue to motivate him and support him. Since going on metformin medicine and eating healthier he hasn't put on any more weight and he has lost 2kg. I feel like there is a light at the end of the tunnel. I'm starting to see a bit of a light.

How much time is enough?

If you visit *Australia's Physical Activity and Sedentary Behaviour Guidelines*,[24] you will see there are very clear recommendations for physical activity for children, adolescents and adults.

These are summarised in the table below.

Age group	Physical activity guidelines
Birth–one year	Supervised, floor-based play in safe environments should be encouraged from birth.
One–five years	Be physically active every day for at least three hours, spread throughout the day.
Five–12 years and 13–17 years	Accumulate at least 60 minutes of moderate to vigorous intensity activity every day. Do a variety of activities and engage in more activity – up to several hours – for additional health benefits.
18–64 years	Accumulate 150–300 minutes (2½–5 hours) of moderate intensity physical activity or 75–150 minutes (1¼–2½ hours) of vigorous intensity physical activity, or an equivalent combination of both moderate and vigorous activities, each week.

Be aware that if you haven't exercised for some time and therefore are not physically fit, your experience of exercise intensity levels will be different to someone who is very fit. For example, if you're overweight and start walking briskly, you may find your heart rate is elevated and you start sweating. Over time as your fitness improves, it will take more than a brisk walk to elevate your heart rate and generate the same physical response.

Make a physical activity plan

Just like your menu plans, having a plan for your weekly activity will ensure it actually happens. Don't wait until you 'have time'. Make your physical activity an appointment with yourself and your family. Just like any other appointment, it must be prioritised and kept. If you have been able to make more time for your health as discussed in stage 3, then there should be an allowance for introducing some form of movement into your week. Experiment with what works for you and your family. Don't forget to have fun!

	PARENT 1		PARENT 2		CHILD 1		CHILD 2		CHILD 3	
	Type/ Intensity	Duration (hours)	Type/ Intensity	Duration (hours)	Type/ Intensity	Duration (hours)	Type/ Intensity	Duration (hours)	Type/ Intensity	Duration (hours)
Monday										
Tuesday										
Wednesday										
Thursday										
Friday										
Saturday AM										
Saturday PM										
Sunday AM										
Sunday PM										

Resources

Check out 10 Ways to Get Moving, below. It will stimulate your thinking about the simple ways you can bring more movement into your life. Try not to overthink it; rather, just get stuck in and start doing it. Be sure to refer to the links in the resources section at the back of the book too. You'll find useful websites and names of organisations with a focus on youth and physical activity, and outdoor family fun and adventure.

Check out this screen time checklist for kids: www.etsy.com/au/listing/697339287/screen-time-checklistkids-printable.

Explore your neighbourhood and find the nearest park, playground, walking and bicycle tracks, beach or indoor and outdoor public swimming pool is. Get in touch with the great local youth-support organisations such as YMCA, PCYC, Scouts and Girl Guides. Just use your imagination and EXPLORE! Or use Google Maps to explore your neighbourhood!

Dr Gary's ten top 10 ways to get your family moving

Starting from easy to harder!

1. Walk or scooter together part or all the way to and from school as many days as you can. Could you take a hillier or more challenging route? I must admit I did this with my children (often without them realising with my so-called 'Daddy short-cuts') but it made them stronger people in mind and body – and developed within them a love of being outdoors and moving.

2. Make a commitment to a fun family weekend activity or adventure – for example a walk or run. The community organisation parkrun Australia runs community Saturday morning 7.30 am fun runs or walks all over Australia and the world (see www.parkrun.com.au). You might only get one or two family members willing to participate initially, perhaps mum and child, but you can encourage other family members by linking the outing with a healthy non-food reward, points to receiving pocket money so your child can save up for a favourite toy, e.g. LEGO or an outing to a theme park! Just talk together around the dinner table about these plans and make a contract! Invite any friends or relatives who want to get more active and fit to support you!

3. Give active toys as presents – perhaps a new soccer ball, cricket bat, running shoes, snorkel, bike or scooter rather than something they do not need or will only use rarely. Link that to a gift to yourself as a parent to go running, walking and cycling!

4. Explore low-cost opportunities for fun physical activity. As I mentioned above, PCYC, YMCA and Scouts are examples, as are other local kids' gymnasium fitness programs. If it is available to you, use the NSW Government Active Kids voucher which contributes $200 per child per year for this specific purpose. When your child is at his or her active session, explore how you as a parent can use this time to do an adult fitness session to show your child how committed you are!

5. Plan ahead for your child's school holidays, so they can be active and outdoors as much as possible, e.g. in a day-camp program where they can meet other children and be active and eat healthily. Pre-pack their lunch and drink (water) if need be to save money and ensure their daily program is not compromised by unhealthy snack food and drinks. This is particularly important over the long summer holidays.

6. Work with your neighbours to see if they have the same challenges with their own children to find time and opportunities to be active, especially over the school holidays. They might be able to share child-minding responsibilities with you.

7. Pokémon GO seems to promote outdoor daily steps and has been effective for many of my clients with autism or ADHD who may not necessarily be able to be involved in team sports or social activities.

8. The app Nature Passport is wonderful to promote outdoor adventures. A client's mother put me on to this and it helped get her inactive child out of the house to explore nature and its beauty. As author Richard Louv stated, 'Nature therapy is both great for the mind, body and soul.'

9. Other active mind activities are all still better than internet games. Utilising the power of art and nature therapy, face painting or ceramic painting, for example, will all help get your kids' minds active, which is a prerequisite to an active body. This includes wonderful mindful colouring books or old-fashioned jigsaw puzzles, which I find most kids and adults love to do!

10. Kids' yoga is an amazing blend of body movement and mindful practice. I would strongly encourage both child and parent to try this if possible. I personally practice Iyengar Yoga, which I think has a wonderful holistic approach aimed at body alignment, mindful breathing and meditation, and setting realistic challenges to improve your practice and living a purposeful life.

But make up your own top ten!

Dr Koala's 50 family fun ways to be active

Can you think about ten of your own to add to the list?

1 Go for a bike ride at your favourite local riding place.

Grab the soccer ball and take the kids to the local park for some goalie practice. **2**

3 Grab the cricket bat and tennis ball to play French cricket.

Go for a nice walk on Sunday to the beach or the local botanic gardens. **4**

5 Climb that local hill to get a great view of the surroundings.

Wake up early and get up to watch the sunrise. **6**

7 Go for a yoga lesson at your local yoga studio – come on Mum, will you go with me?

Practice some ball throwing to see who can throw the furthest. **8**

9 Play a game of backyard cricket with the kids.

Go for a walk with your partner and hold each other's hands. **10**

11 Get outside on the trampoline for some lumpy jumpy days.

Take the dog for a walk and don't forget his favourite ball. **12**

13 Join your local parkrun for 5km walk or run and make some new friends.

Grab the boxing gloves and give Dad a good session. **14**

15 Take up photography

16 Let's practice 25m sprints in the local park! Who can be the fastest?

17 It's summer so let's grab the boogie board and hit the waves!

18 Let's do some diving at the local diving pool!

19 Wow, let's go shell hunting in the shallows at the rocks at the beach.

20 Can we monkey bar from one end to the other?

21 I love the see-saw and the merry-go-round and climbing ropes at my local park.

22 Grab your skipping rope and see how many times you can skip without stopping.

23 Hip hop music is my favourite to dance to! Let's move!

24 Can you do a handstand or cartwheel yet?

25 Let's grab the football and do some kick passing to each other at the park.

26 I would love to try rock climbing at the local indoor climbing studio!

27 What about a spin cycle session at the local gym?

28 YMCA has a great Uplift program for 12 years old and above! Let's go!

29 I love mixed martial arts at the PCYC.

30 Fencing can be fun – wow, I feel like a musketeer!

31 What about space walking? Let's pretend we are in outer space!

32 Can we pretend we are in the Olympics and in the 100m relay team? Where is our baton? Maybe we can make paper ones! And the four of us can run around the oval.

33 Why don't we climb up all those stairs at the local dam?

34 Let's walk backwards at the park and try not to fall over?

35 Can we play piggyback races with Dad and Mum?

36 Wow I have never played golf before but it looks like fun. Can we go to the golfing range to try it out?

37 I do love table tennis. Is there a local table tennis centre nearby we can play at?

38 Can we shoot a few baskets at the local school, Dad? I need to improve my free throws!

39 Let's go mountain bike riding this weekend down that new trail.

40 Wouldn't it be fun to join the Scouts and do some camping overnight, Dad and Mum?

41 I want to be a Karate Kid and fly!

42 Can we ride our bikes to school, please Mum?

43 I love Wet 'n' Wild – that water slide is so big and scary but so much fun! Can we go, Mum?

44 I love to catch the ferry to Manly or Circular Quay, Dad. Can we go this weekend for fun outing?

45 The zoo is great, Dad. I love the tigers and the way they move, and the koalas are so cute!

46 Wouldn't it be nice if we could go for a beach holiday, Dad?

47 Could I learn to play tennis, Dad? It looks like fun.

48 Dad, can you teach me how to ride a bike? I think I am old enough now!

49 My friend wants me to go the YMCA gym with them to do some cardio. Can we go? You might enjoy the adult sessions.

50 I love Zumba classes – the music makes me want to move!

Notes

....

....

....

....

....

....

....

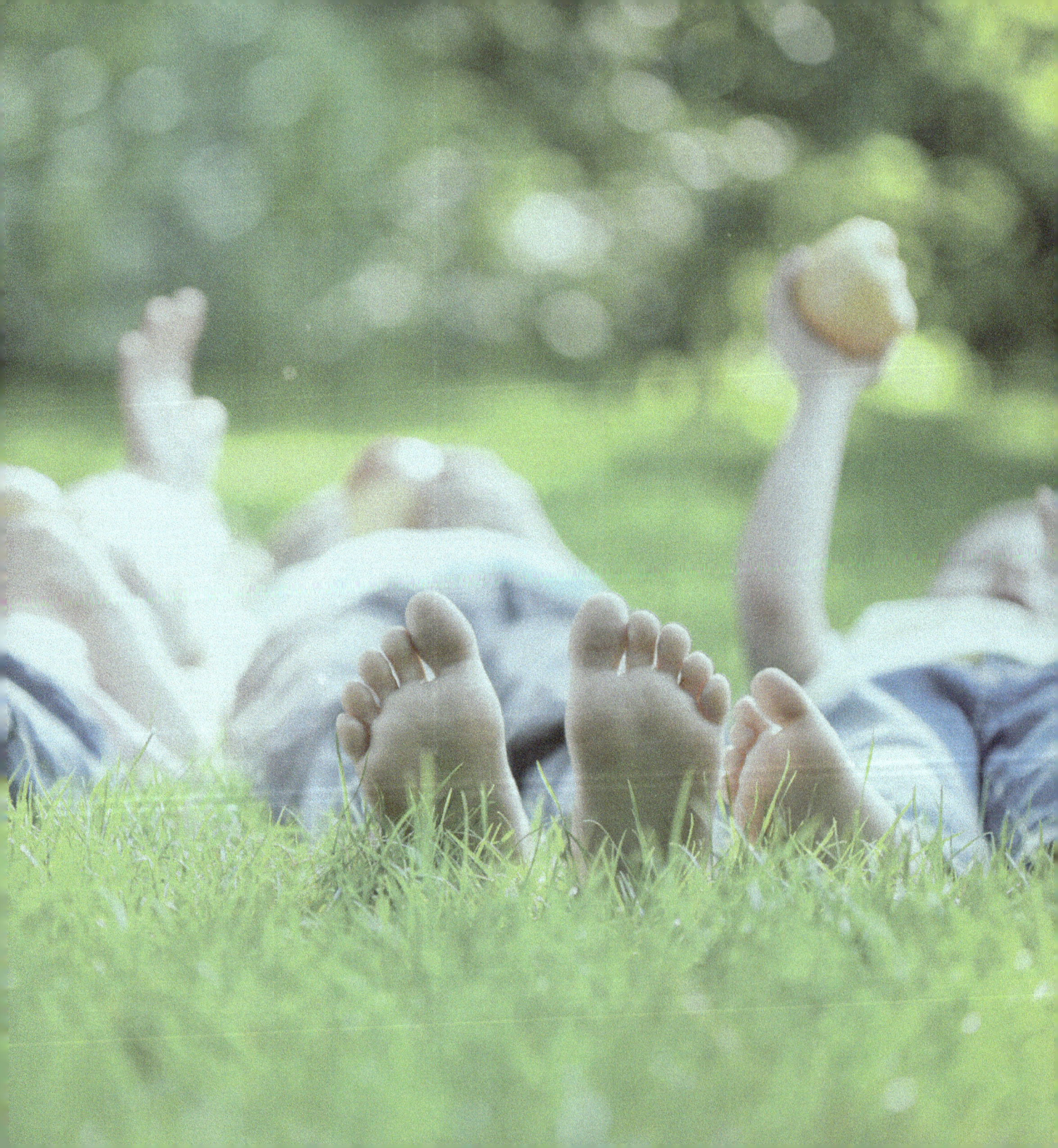

Stage 7

Sleep, Problematic Internet Use (PIU) and its effects on cognitive function and mental and physical health

I can think. I can sleep. I can move. I can ride my bike. I can dream.

Bill Walton, American athlete

Sleep is the Swiss army knife of health. When sleep is deficient, there is sickness and disease. And when sleep is abundant, there is vitality and health.

Matthew Walker, Neuroscientist and author of Why We Sleep.

In this stage, which focuses on sleep, we will:

- Highlight the mental and physical health benefits of good sleep.
- Explain the damaging effects caused by poor sleep.
- Give guidance for how to get the whole family sleeping well.
- Explore how excessive screen time, especially in regards to internet gaming in adolescence, has crept up on parents over the last 10 years.

Excessive screen time is causing havoc with developing mental and physical health, with behaviours linked with obesity around poor sleep, overeating, sedentariness and withdrawal from physical activity and normal healthy family and social relationships.

How much sleep do you and your children get each weeknight and on the weekends?

You might like to do this little exercise over a typical week during school term and write down the time you get to bed and then when you actually get to sleep for each individual in your family.

For an adult sleep diary see this one from the National Sleep Foundation: www.sleepfoundation.org/sites/default/files/inline-files/SleepDiaryv6.pdf

One more suitable for your child from the National Sleep Foundation is available here: www.sleepforkids.org/pdf/SleepDiary.pdf

You may not be surprised that either yourself or most of your children are not getting the recommended number of hours of sleep.

This is what is recommended by the National Sleep Foundation in the USA based on a rigorous review of the scientific literature.

Sleep duration recommendations:

As a rough guide, pre-schoolers should be aiming for 10–13 hours sleep a night, primary school children should be getting about 10 hours and older children at least nine hours, while adults should aim for eight hours a night.

Age	Recommended	May be appropriate	Not recommended
Newborns 0–3 months	14–17 hours	11–13 hours 18–19 hours	Less than 11 hours More than 19 hours
Infants 4–11 months	12–15 hours	10–11 hours 16–18 hours	Less than 10 hours More than 18 hours
Toddlers 1–2 years	11–14 hours	9–10 hours 15–16 hours	Less than 9 hours More than 16 hours
Preschoolers 3–5 years	10–13 hours	8–9 hours 14 hours	Less than 8 hours More than 14 hours
Young school-aged Children 6–13 years	9–11 hours	7–8 hours 12 hours	Less than 7 hours More than 12 hours
Teenagers 14–17 years	8–10 hours	7 hours 11 hours	Less than 7 hours More than 11 hours

Age	Recommended	May be appropriate	Not recommended
Young Adults 18–25 years	7–9 hours	6 hours 10–11 hours	Less than 6 hours More than 11 hours
Adults 26–64 years	7–9 hours	6 hours 10 hours	Less than 6 hours More than 10 hours
Older Adults ≥ 65 years	7–8 hours	5–6 hours 9 hours	Less than 5 hours More than 9 hours

Good luck with that!

Numerous studies have shown an association between lack of sleep and increased risk for obesity, diabetes and high blood pressure. This begs the question, what is the actual function of sleep for our bodies? We all know that feeling after having a few late nights out or working late or studying for an exam. We know how our body automatically tells us through tiredness and sleepiness that we need to catch up on the lost hours of sleep, usually at the weekend!

However, sleep deprivation has other profound effects on your bodily functions that impact negatively on your risk for obesity, mental health and many other disorders. The fact is that in the modern Western world sleep deprivation has now been declared an epidemic (WHO – 'Sleepless in America', as shown on National Geographic: www.nih.gov/news-events/news-releases/nih-research-featured-national-geographic-channel-documentary-sleep).

Sleep deprivation has been linked to the following health problems:

- Depression and anxiety[25]
- Disordered immune function and inflammation, including risk for cancer.
- Obesity and diabetes, through effects on appetite and blood glucose levels.
- Cardiovascular disease, including high blood pressure.
- Accidents at work or while driving.
- Memory impairment, including risk for from dementia!

Tragically, there are more and more cases of children and teenagers who do no exercise at all, spending far too much time being sedentary on their technology of some form. Lack of exercise combined with too much time on technology is having a devastating effect on children's sleep cycles, causing their metabolism to be disrupted, which in turn aggravates the cycle of obesity.

It really is just a vicious and sickening cycle that contributes further to obesity and other associated conditions, including anxiety and depression.

In addition, the powerful brain-maturing effects of adequate deep sleep during the teenage years are essential for frontal-lobe maturation and rationality to flourish.[26] This difference in brain maturation in adolescents is associated with an altered circadian rhythm and explains why it is so hard to get your teenage child off to bed early and why it is so hard to get them up early as well! Some secondary schools have recognised the inherent differences in teenage brains and sleep cycles, and have deliberately moved school start times an hour or so later for teenagers!

Healthy Sleep Tips

I give this Happy Sleep Habits sheet to my clients in the clinic: www.actionforhappiness.org/media/655415/50_ways_download_-_happy_sleep_habits.pdf

It emphasises the following:

- Make a regular, routine bed and sleep time.
- Withdraw any technology at least one–two hours before this time.
- Have a glass of milk before bed and before you brush your teeth – the latter is my suggestion to ensure healthy teeth!
- Make the room sufficiently dark with no TV, phone or computer in the room to disturb those dreams!
- It is also important to make sure the room is not too warm; in fact, a cool 18 degrees is best as once you are under the sheets and doona (in winter) you will warm up! And the body naturally lowers its temperature at night to prepare for sleep.

Problematic Internet Use (PIU)

In my practice, the typical teenager I see is up late at night or having 'all-nighters' on technology and gaming. Often the games they are playing are violent and inappropriate for their age. More than contributing to poor sleep quality and habits, these behaviours are destructive in other ways. Their day/night cycle is disrupted, which in turn affects normal sleep patterns. The flow on effect from this is raised cortisol hormone levels, which then promote hunger and fat production in the body. A terrible negative cycle, the teenager gains weight and becomes even more sedentary due to the increasing physical difficulty of carrying the excessive weight. They are less amenable to the idea of breaking the cycle because it just feels all too hard. Sadly, this pattern is being repeated in households all over the world. What's worse is that it's avoidable if parents and their children start owning their share of responsibility for their respective lives.

I have seen many examples of teenage children suffering from a combination of lack of sleep, screen addiction, spending countless hours on the internet, gaming anxiety and school truancy. Commonly, these adolescent boys, more often than not, are addicted to these online games, e.g. Fortnite and other more violent ones that are specifically designed to exploit the reward systems in our brain, just like the design of poker machines!

What is the effect of this screen and gaming addiction? Apart from significantly reducing sleep quantity, it creates in the adolescent an alteration of the natural sleep phase through interference of dark–light/sleep–wake cycles. Typically, this ends up leading the adolescent to stay awake gaming well into the night and early morning, and then makes them unable to wake until after noon! And while this may be sustainable during school holidays, it is not during school terms. Sleep deprivation alone alters cognitive function and the ability to store memories, and will inevitably interfere with school performance, coping with everyday stress and the desire to be physically active or make healthy food choices.

Brad Marshall, the Unplugged Psychologist, is the author of *The Tech Diet for your Child & Teen*. Brad has one of the few internet addiction clinics in Australia at Northshore Kidspace in Chatswood, Sydney. He describes a series of symptoms and behaviours below that might suggest that your child's internet usage is becoming problematic and that he or she should perhaps seek advice and help.

Signs of internet addiction:

- neglecting school, university or work
- loss or withdrawal of social interaction in favour of online platforms
- neglecting regular sleep or eating patterns to stay online
- being dishonest with others about online use
- feeling anxious, angry, depressed or angry as a result of online behaviour
- withdrawal from other activities like sport
- feeling irritable or moody with angry outbursts when asked to come offline
- internet use causing arguments within families.

These problematic behaviours that arise from the excessive screen time have an ill effect on sleep health and in turn on mood, and lead to behaviours that cause obesity, such as overeating, unhealthy snacking, and lack of regular daily physical activity and normal healthy social interaction. There is also an effect on family relationships between the child and his or her parents and siblings.

It is beyond this book and the Ride to Life program to adequately help you if you recognise your child has an internet addiction problem. It goes without saying that you need to seek help, either from Dr Brad Marshall's book or a local clinical psychologist who has experience with treating children with internet addiction.

Be aware that as a parent that you may need to first address your own relationship with the internet and examine how healthy your own use of this essential modern tool is before helping your own child.

Remember the one rule for all and all for one philosophy. Restricting your child's internet or screen time is of course going to elicit an unfavourable, negative reaction, but talk this through with your child. Ask them if they feel it is a problem and how their use of the internet is affecting their relationships with school, friends, family and their community. And as Dr Brad outlines in his book, negotiate a contract that all parties can hopefully agree to, and adopt the attitude that the internet is a reward not a right! It has to be earned with certain teenage-appropriate responsibilities around the house. For example, keeping their room clean and tidy, eating with the family and not alone in their room, or regular daily physical activity. I like this last one particularly; as an example, you might agree to one hour of internet for every hour of physical activity during the week, but then you have to provide that opportunity to be active with your teenager!

Negative reactions from your child and teenager like verbal abuse and physical abuse cannot be tolerated and should come with consequences, such as removal of access to internet completely for 24–48 hours to allow your child to reflect on their behaviour.

To be honest, there is no magic answer to this very common problem. You as the parent have to do the best you can, try to be fair and keep the lines of communication open, and when you are in trouble and not making progress seek some professional help.

Gently try to get your child to develop their own insight into how this internet addiction is a problem and explore with them the possible solutions. At all times stay calm and if the first conversation about this does not work then try again. Don't give up – this is too important for the health of the whole family. This may include making a commitment to getting more physical activity at set times of the day after school or on the weekends with you to minimise the time available for internet use.

Try remember the three 'L's for happier families: love, limits and laughter! In the end as the parent you sometimes have to take control and make a decision for them that limits their internet time though restricting access via a password or by linking access to positive behaviour, e.g. physical activity and acceptable behaviour.

Resources

Make sure you also get across to the Ride to Life website and access all the online resources that are available there.

Professor Matthew Walker, Professor of Neuroscience at University of California, Berkeley, USA has several interesting videos, including a TED Talk, to accompany his book *Why We Sleep*: www.sleepdiplomat.com/speaker

National Science Foundation (USA) has some great resources, including tips and a sleep diary: www.sleepfoundation.org/sleep-solutions/sleep-tools-tips

Brad Marshall, *The Tech Diet for your Child & Teen*, 2019: www.unpluggedpsychologist.com

If you need more information in this area of ongoing research, Dr Phillip Tam is a child and adolescent psychiatrist in Sydney and his website is helpful: www.thedeltaclinic.com.au

Network for Internet Investigation and Research Australia: www.niira.org.au/

Dr Michael Mosley, medical doctor, science journalist and author of several important health-related books, including *The Fast Diet, The Fast 800* and *The Clever Guts Diet*, has just released his latest book, *Fast Asleep*. Michael's new book explains how to get better sleep and cure insomnia. Dr K needs to read this one for sure, as do many of you.

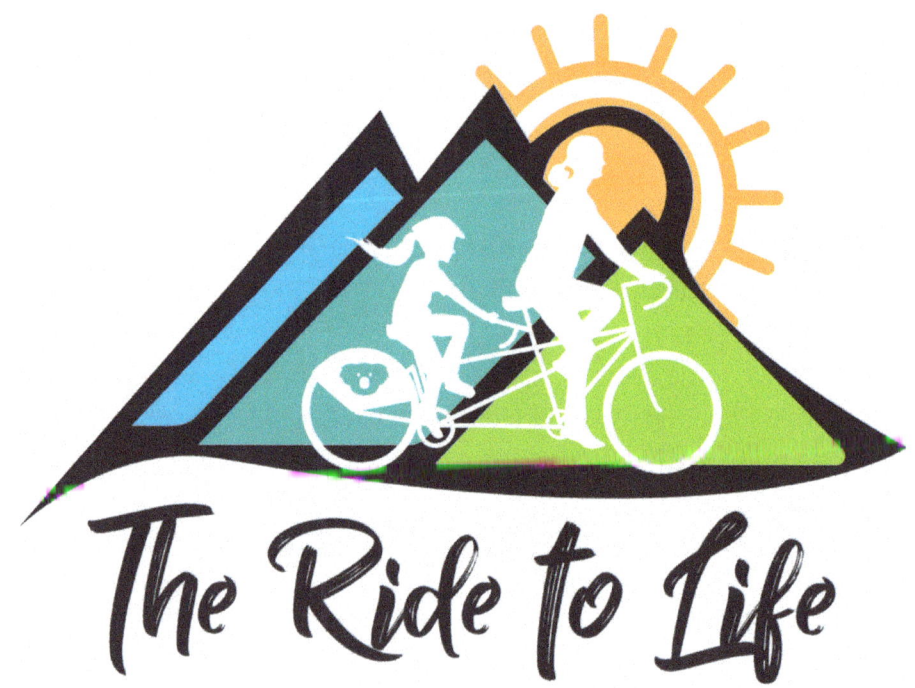

PARTIE 3
ON THE ROAD

In training and doing the hard yards

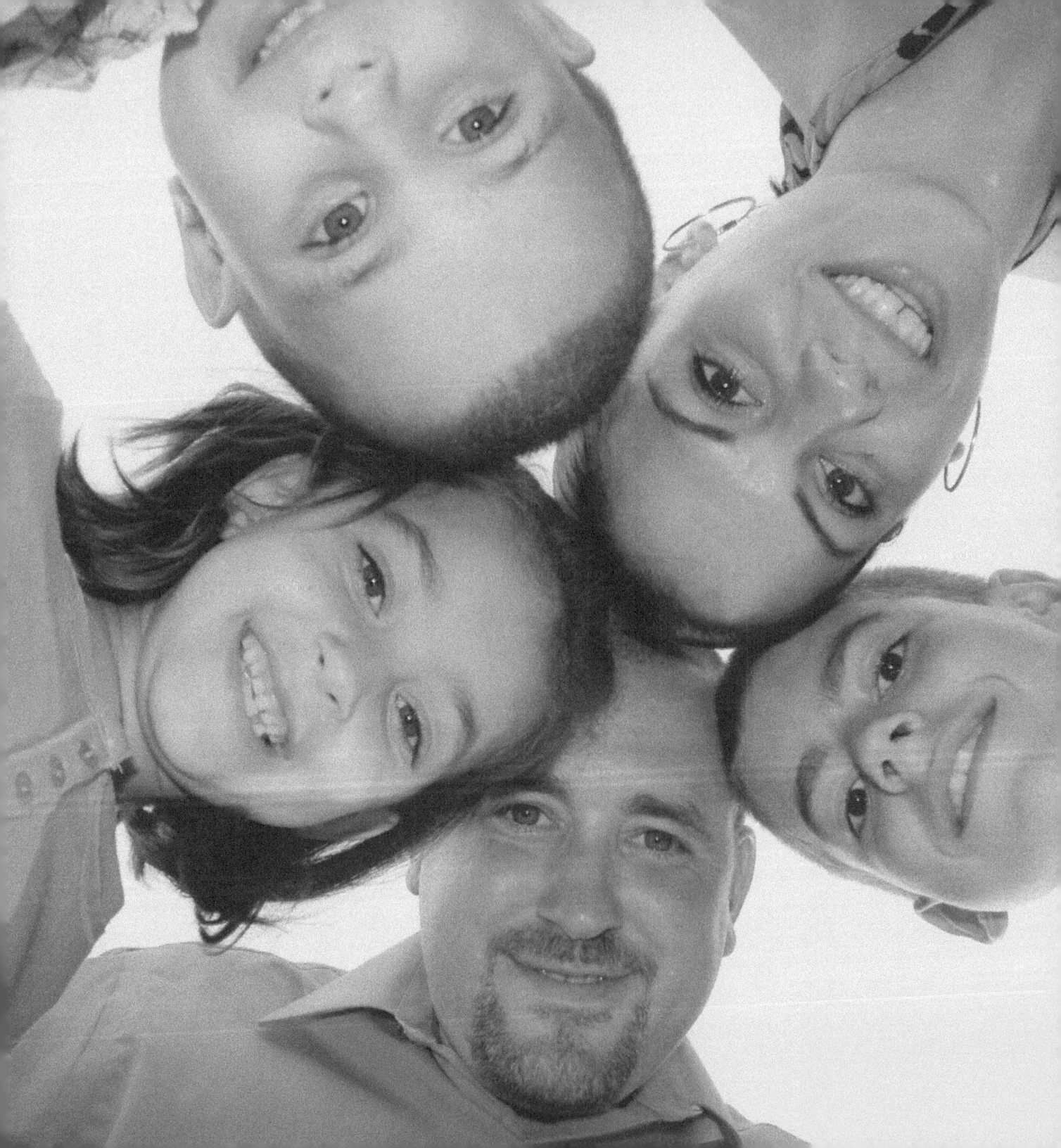

Stage 8

Connection, self-care and support

> *Your body is the child of the soul. You must nourish and train your child.*
>
> Sri B.K.S. Iyengar, Yogi and Founder of Iyengar School of Yoga

In this stage, we will:

- Outline the importance and benefits of having a strong, reliable support structure in place.
- Learn about the 'disconnection syndrome'.
- Identify the ideal people to provide support and encouragement without judgement.
- Learn the importance of nurturing these support relationships in a healthy way, such that it benefits both you and the support person.

Having a healthy life means getting connected

A common experience I witness with most patients in my clinic is the absence of healthy human connections in their lives. Applying to parents, grandparents, and a broader social circle, it's just another indicator of disconnection. Frankly, it saddens me people feel more isolated from each other than they've ever been. I see this phenomenon so often, sometimes described by the term 'the disconnection syndrome'. In fact, when I first thought about writing this book several years ago, I considered using this as the title. It has since been taken up by several authors in the social-research field including Johann Hari in his insightful book *Lost Connections: Uncovering the Real Cause Of Depression – And The Unexpected Solutions* and, of course: Richard Louv in his book *The Nature Principle: Reconnecting with Life in a Virtual Age*.

The disconnection syndrome

The disconnection syndrome is a contemporary epidemic that is noticeably prevalent in Western society but spreading across the globe. Despite increased digital connectivity enjoyed via technology, conversely and increasingly, we are more disconnected from the very things that contribute to our overall health and wellbeing in physical, mental and spiritual terms.

This is based on the premise that the more connected you are with yourself (as a person), within the family (whatever that represents for you), community, nature ('the nature principle'), your food and food sources, and your personal vision/dreams for the future (purpose), the more likely you are to make wise choices for your health and the health of your children.

Equally, the more disconnected you are with these spheres of life, the greater the likelihood you will find yourself on the chronic-disease trajectory, suffering from obesity, type 2 diabetes, and heart disease. This disconnection is also inextricably linked to mental illnesses like anxiety and depression.

Families who typically suffer from the disconnection syndrome often display these symptoms:

- Chronically stressed.
- Time-poor and without a regular, manageable routine in any area of life.
- Feel a lack of control in their lives.
- Can't see a vision for a different, improved, healthier life.

Families who are connected, stay healthy and thriving display different characteristics. Family members, including extended family, are likely to demonstrate the following behaviours:

- Share similar values, give the same healthy messages, and are consistent with children in terms of boundaries and behavioural expectations.
- Share responsibilities in the day-to-day activities of the family, considering each person's contributions to the health and wellbeing of the family.
- Parents prioritise their self-care, with the realisation that as leaders in the family, they must care for themselves so they provide the same level of care to children from a full, rather than depleted, cup.
- Can manage stress without it negatively impacting the family's life.
- Enjoy established and manageable routines that provide a healthy sense of control over their lives.
- Have a vision for their future and see it unfolding.

Connection starts with you

It's easy to see how we're disconnected from the external world, but what about internally? Aren't we disconnected there, too?

In my opinion, we have never been more disconnected from ourselves. Just look at the global epidemic of obesity. From a mental/emotional perspective, obesity represents disconnection from ourselves. No doubt, there are genetic, physical and other aspects to obesity, but there are also the emotional and mental aspects too. My opinion may upset some of my medical and scientific colleagues, but we cannot hope to address obesity in anyone, let alone in our children, if we do not make the emotional and spiritual aspects a primary consideration in any treatment solutions. In practical terms, if we are to have any hope of correcting this, we need to make reconnecting with ourselves one of our highest priorities.

In my clinic, I commonly hear from mothers that they do not take time to nurture themselves. The challenge of caring for a family, balancing work and other commitments, and negotiating relationship parameters (including with your partner) can be overwhelming. Add to this the (often misplaced) external social pressures that urge us to keep doing/having more means many parents and primary caregivers end up putting their own needs last. A recipe for disaster, this approach only serves to perpetuate the cycle of obesity. More so than men, women are socialised to be carers, often putting others before themselves.

As a parent – irrespective of whether you're a mum, dad, guardian or carer – your own self-care is your responsibility and it needs to be your highest priority.

Only when you take care of yourself, are you better equipped to do the following:

- Withstand judgement from anyone (family, friends and professionals included) who questions your parenting ability in the face of a child with obesity.
- Hold firm to boundaries that need to established and maintained when implementing healthier behaviours in your family.
- Support your child as they integrate the new behaviours and foods into their life.
- Remember your '**Why**' for this journey.
- Ride out the tough and low days when things seem too hard and you feel like giving up.

It takes time, experimentation, patience and persistence to develop this self-care muscle and to get these things right. Until this muscle develops, recognise that sometimes it will be a case of two steps forward and one step back. Fortunately, there will always be challenges that arise, providing opportunities to refine your approach, and reorient yourself and the family. Through diligent self-care practices, you give yourself the best chance of staying on track. I encourage you to become more comfortable with the idea that self-care is another important and essential strategy in your tool box for reclaiming life and breaking the cycle of obesity in your family.

 ## Starting with self-care

Take a few minutes to reflect what self-care means to you. Looking after ourselves in healthy ways, after spending many years doing the opposite, is about learning and committing to new behaviours.

Write down five things you can have as go-to activities for self-care:

1.

2.

3.

4.

5.

Once you've listed these five things, commit to doing one regularly, at least every week, or more often if possible. Remember, it doesn't need to be expensive. It could be as simple as buying yourself a nice bunch of flowers, watching your favourite movie or TV show uninterrupted, having a soothing aromatherapy bath, getting a massage, having a coffee or herbal tea by yourself without the kids, listening to some music you love or taking a 30-minute walk in nature without any other distractions. If you've reviewed your family's routine and been able to make time and space for change, hopefully there is some time in your week to spend on nurturing yourself. Remember you are helping everyone when you help yourself, so commit to it.

Understanding the family dynamic

When families first come to see me in the clinic, I ask them draw up a family tree. Doing this provides very useful insights to the current family dynamic. It also sheds light on the origin of these inter-generational issues.

I have the parent draw a family tree outlining the various family members and the level of support each member is perceived to provide, including the grandparents, aunts, uncles and cousins on both sides of the family. And that's exactly what we're going to do now.

Reflect on your own family

Complete this exercise using the instructions below. I also suggest doing it at a time when you know you won't be interrupted or distracted as the exercise requires absolute honesty and some of the insights could be quite emotional for you.

Start by drawing your immediate family (you and your partner, if you have one, and the kids) and then scale out to include other generations and branches. Every family is different: some have two parents with two kids, while others have solo parents or carers, some are blended or have same-sex parents. The composition of your family though important, is not critical for this exercise.

What we're interested in here is the quality of the relationships and connections you have with people you consider family.

As you draw up the tree, make notes about the nature of the relationships between the family members. For instance, is there tension between you and another family member? Do two members of your family often clash? Are any members of your family not speaking to other members?

Next, identify the health of each family member, including whether they are suffering, or have suffered, from a range of health conditions, including obesity, diabetes, heart or liver disease, stroke, high blood pressure, cholesterol problems or cancer. It is important, though challenging, to highlight if there is a family history of drug abuse, alcohol abuse, smoking or other addictions, or family violence.

Next, rate each member in your family in terms of their likely level of support in your endeavours to improve the quality of health of your family. Use the following support score scale:

0 – Not at all supportive/don't know   1 – Somewhat supportive   2 – Fully supportive

> The value of this exercise is in how it provides a pointer to who within your family is likely to support your efforts on this important journey. On reflection, if you find there are very few or no family members that you feel will readily support you, don't despair; there will be people outside your family who will. Even if you don't know who they are yet, that's OK. We'll get to that.
>
> I encourage you to do this exercise honestly. These considerations are common drivers of the cycle of obesity and you may have already recognised the way these family factors have contributed to your own situation. Reaching this level of honesty is not easy, so if you have been willing to do this, keep going. It will give insights into you and your family, allowing you to break free from the cycle of obesity.

Who's got your back

Because this journey is tough, you cannot afford to have people on your team who haven't got your back 100 percent. Teamwork is so important in everything in life. It's the same in sport too. In Le Tour de France, there is a close bond between members within a cycling team. Each rider in the team has a role to play and the team itself is supported by a virtual army of chefs, physiotherapists, doctors, massage therapists and coaches. It is only through the teamwork of *every* member, including the non-cycling members, that success is even possible.

Success in creating real and lasting change for your family also depends on assembling an effective and cohesive team. You must also have people who are fully supportive of your commitment to a healthier, happier life. When preparing the family tree, you will have an opportunity to note names of any family members who scored at least a three. These people *may* be the first people to go to for support. However, be aware not everybody will be supportive of your desire to be healthier. Anyone who didn't score above two in your assessment should be remain off your list until they demonstrate a willingness to support you. Know that while their support may not be forthcoming immediately, it may come in time. Also, be conscious that as you change the dynamic within your family will also change. As a result, you might find support comes from surprising and unexpected avenues.

I present this concept of the support team here to highlight areas in which your own family might not be functioning in the best way to support the changes you want to make for yourself, your child and your family.

Resistance from family

Be aware, as you strive to break the cycle of obesity, it may lead to unexpected changes in your relationships (opposition, dismissal, anger or hopefully positive changes including acceptance, support and love for you putting your family's health so high on your priority list), adding another dimension of complexity to the journey. I often see people in my clinic whose partner or child's grandparents are not supportive.

Resistance can come in many different forms to any changes you try to implement. It might be as simple as totally ignoring your wishes to stop bringing so much junk food into the house as presents, or grandparents having junk food around when your child visits, or even their father deliberately ignoring your wishes when he picks them up from school, still driving through McDonald's when he knows you are trying to instill some healthy changes.

This will frustrate you, scare you and may lead to a situation where you need to confront your spouse or parents or parents-in-law. How you deal with confrontation will be the key if you are to overcome this roadblock. You need to be clear in your own mind why *you* think this is important and express this clearly and calmly to your spouse or your parents. *They need to know this is unacceptable* and that they need to be accountable for their actions in working against your expressed wishes. Are you ready to face such a confrontation for the health of your child? If you know your '**Why**' then you should be able to keep strong and stick to your goal, but it will not be easy.

Relationships are the most difficult thing to develop and nurture. If they wander along with neither party happy then sadly it might be time to ask yourself if it is worth it – and then, what is the alternative? This is a very difficult question many couples do not have the courage to ask themselves.

I am not sure I want to be a marriage or relationship counsellor, but we are talking about the health and wellbeing of *your* child. All who play a major role in your child's life need to stand up, take some care and responsibility, and be accountable for their actions or inactions. It is that simple, really!

Going outside the family for support

In my clinical experience, it is essential to look outside your family for support. The reality is family brings conditions and conditioning that in part has contributed to your current situation, either directly or indirectly. For this reason, it is healthy and wise to seek external support from other sources.

Instinctively, we think our closest friends will be the providers of that support. While this might be true, there is also a possibility your friends may resist your changes, particularly if they are also living in the cycle of obesity. I say this because we frequently socialise with those who reflect our values. In this instance, I can refer to a specific study which highlighted that the most important relationships contributing to the cycle of obesity are those with our closest friends. That's right, our best friends![27] Because these relationships are often long-standing, we must navigate carefully through the process of identifying external support people, while also managing the changes in current relationships brought about by new and healthier ways of living.

People you'd approach for support include those with the following characteristics:

- Are accepting and non-judgemental. They understand that we all experience life challenges in one form or another and accept you for who you are and what you are trying to achieve.
- Are supportive and encouraging, but call you higher (this means you behave within your values and purpose) when you want to take the easy option.
- Have a capacity for listening. They don't just talk about themselves, but are open to hearing your deepest concerns, fears and dreams on your Ride to Life.
- Demonstrate unwavering integrity. They will do the right thing by you, even if that means challenging you.
- Are dependable and reliable, i.e. they do what they say they will.
- Are honest, steadfast, consistent and respectful.

Now you know *what* to look for, can you think of anyone in your network who fits the bill? Make a note of them below and keep adding to the list over time. The key here is not quantity, it's quality. The process of choosing people is about being conscious of who to include in your support team.

From a personal perspective, support may come from any of the following:

- Social and sporting clubs and gyms you may choose to join
- Religious or spiritual groups
- Work colleagues
- Community groups
- Support groups, on and offline.

 **Make your list**

Write down the names of people (family and non-family members) on your support crew here. Also make a note of the area in which they provide support.

The key people on my support crew list are:

1.
Support provided:

2.
Support provided:

3.
Support provided:

Keep adding to this list over time.

What if you're having trouble identifying suitable people to add to your support crew?

Please don't be disheartened. The right support will appear at the right time. Just by opening your mind to the idea that you need quality people supporting you, the space is created for these people to appear.

As a start, you can join the Ride to Life support team. An online social support network, it will provide connection with like-minded people who are committed to breaking the cycle of obesity and creating a healthier, happier life.

Support can also be drawn from inspirational people and stories. For example, TED Talks offer up some wonderful insights into all kinds of topics and are free to view. These can be sourced through your local library and online. For me, I find inspiration from understanding the stories behind other people's struggles for health, happiness and freedom. It reminds me that although our challenges may be individual, the experience of overcoming them and growing through them is universal. Without exception, our challenges provide the greatest opportunity for us to grow. Remember, there is always someone worse off than you. While it may seem like I'm minimising the challenges you face, as I say to my patients in the clinic, now is the time to count your blessings, not your calories.

What about medical support?

Although I am a medically trained doctor, I am disappointed by the level and quality of support given by most health professionals to people suffering from the effects of obesity. Unfortunately, I've observed this in medical doctors more than I'd like, who, in the treatment of chronic conditions like obesity, are frequently lacking in empathy.

While I'm not excusing this unpleasant treatment towards patients, medical training doesn't equip a 21st century medical practitioner with the required knowledge and skills to address the greatest medical public health problem facing the globe, i.e. obesity and related chronic disease.[28] However, having the support of an empathetic medical professional is a wise move and you may seek help from one or a number of the following:

- Your general practitioner and paediatrician.
- Specialists, such as a general physician, endocrinologist or psychiatrist.
- Allied health professionals, such as an experienced dietician, exercise physiologist, psychologist, physiotherapist, nurse or diabetes educator.
- Some alternative therapists, including massage therapists, yoga and mindfulness teachers.
- Seeking a second opinion or alternative primary heath team.

I provide the following caveat for alternative therapists: if you choose alternative therapies, particularly at the early stage of your journey, do so with the understanding that it's essential to adopt an integrated approach with Western medicine. This means bringing together the different ways of doing things, including both medical treatment (which, in many cases is necessary for keeping people with acute conditions well) and alternative therapies. If you don't approach treatment for your child's condition in this way, you are at risk of exposing the child and yourself to unnecessary stress, potentially making things worse. A sensible and balanced approach is what's required.

By becoming part of the Ride to Life Program, you can share and read inspirational stories of others who are on the same journey and facing the same struggles. Equally, there will be others who have reached a healthier, happier destination and can keep you focused on where you want to take your family's health.

Resources

Make sure you also get across to the Ride to Life website and access all the online resources that are available there.

Author and journalist, Johann Hari has published a book called *Lost Connections: Uncovering the Real Causes of Depression – and the Unexpected Solutions*.[29] Johann's book is well worth a read if you are curious about the connection between how you feel and what you do.

Notes

....

....

....

....

....

....

....

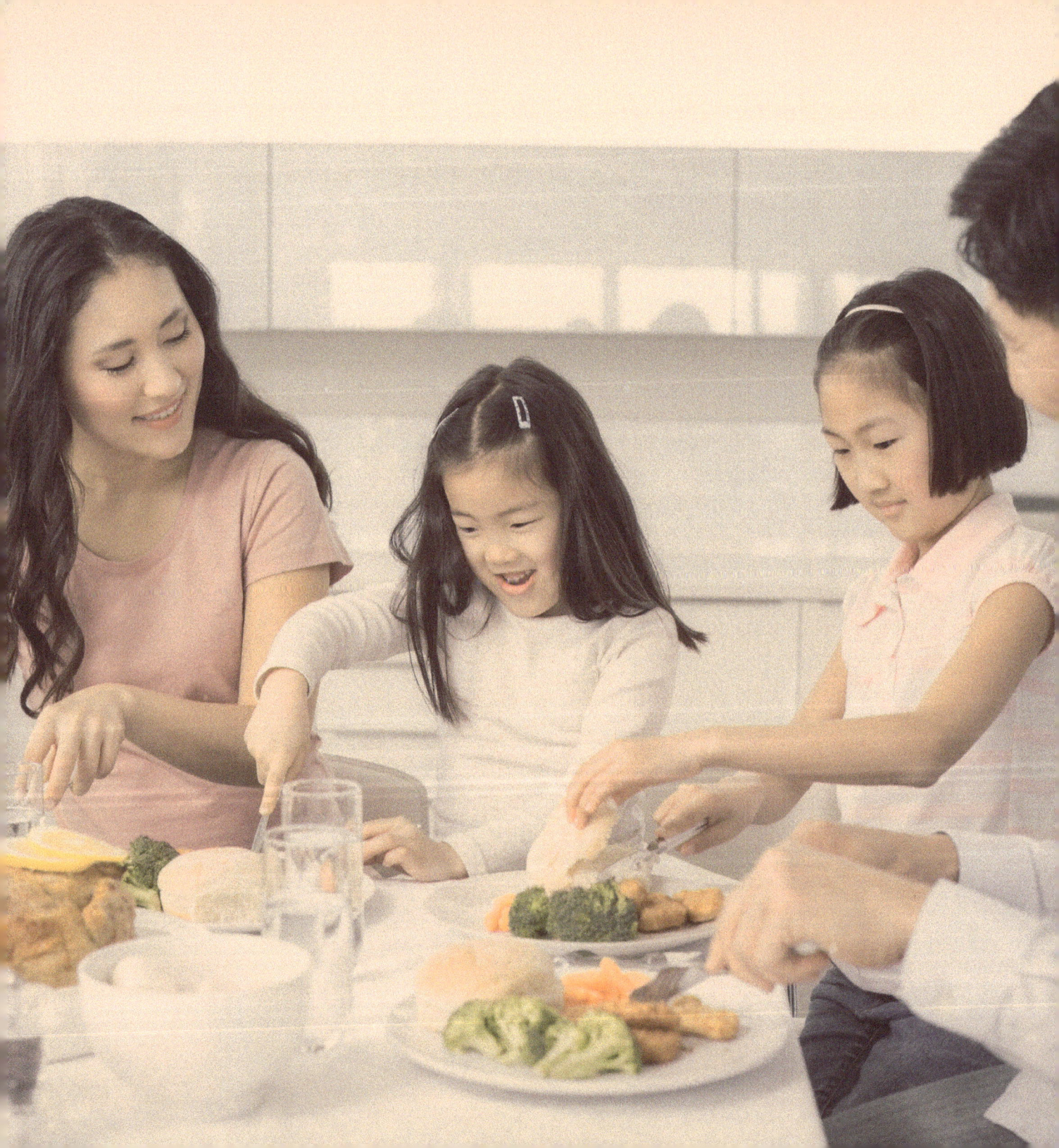

Stage 9

The power of 'no': why you need it and how to use it.

> *When you take charge of your life, there is no longer need to ask permission of other people or society at large. When you ask permission, you give someone veto power over your life.*
>
> Geoffrey F. Abert, US author, 1970

I have come to understand the importance of boundaries through my friend Roslyn Saunders. Roslyn is the author of the book *Emotional Sobriety: Finding Raw Courage to Recover from Co-dependency* and the founder of an online support group called Power of No. She is a co-dependency recovery coach and is the best person I know for learning how to set and hold firm to boundaries in relationships. With her permission, the content in this stage is referenced directly from her book and adapted to the context of addressing the cycle of obesity.

In this stage, we will:

- Outline the importance of boundaries and why they're necessary for breaking the cycle of obesity and creating a healthier, happier life.
- Learn how to set boundaries and hold firm to them.

Before I met Roslyn, I didn't understand the concept of co-dependency (I didn't even know the meaning of the word), but through her teaching I've come to understand co-dependency is the 'disease' of the lost self.[30] In simple terms, this means when we're disconnected from ourselves, we don't make choices for our highest good. Poor decisions are reflected in our mental, emotional and physical health, and our wellbeing. And until we identify what we need, we can't make those good choices. What you'll discover in this stage is when those needs are identified, it's necessary to bring the power of 'no' into your life.

In *Emotional Sobriety*, Roslyn writes:

> Co-dependence is the condition of low self-esteem – the lost self – wherein we have difficulty making decisions. We value others' approval, thinking, feelings and behaviour over our own.

Affecting all of us at some level, I feel this is relevant for any parent whose child is living with obesity because we're unable to say no and hold firm to it. We've also taught our children they can't say no either. I've found this to be true through my own clinical practice when I talk with parents. So many of them tell me they just can't say no to their child.

Developing boundaries

Answer the questions below to gain insights into your own co-dependency.

Just as you have with every other aspect of your journey to break the cycle of obesity, this exercise requires honesty and courage. Instead of seeing it as a chore or challenge, think of it as another important step towards strengthening the resolve that will help break the cycle of obesity in your family.

I set limits on food intake and items, but I find it difficult to remain committed to these.	☐ True ☐ False
I feel shame and guilt because I have a child who is living with obesity and I end up covering over these feelings with food (eating too much/eating junk foods or not eating enough).	☐ True ☐ False
When I'm in stressful situations, my go-to strategy is to eat for comfort.	☐ True ☐ False
I have moments where I feel things have gone too far, and then I think what's the point of even trying to create a healthier life for me and my child.	☐ True ☐ False
I allow my child or partner (and others) to abuse me when I say no and attempt to hold firm to a boundary.	☐ True ☐ False
When I'm in a social setting, such as an event, party or family gathering, my resolve about food boundaries dissolves, i.e. I give in to a boundary I've set.	☐ True ☐ False
I feel pressured to attend social events with family or friends and consume food or drinks that I know aren't healthy for me or my family.	☐ True ☐ False
I feel my needs are always at the bottom of the list and never seem to be taken care of.	☐ True ☐ False
I feel like I've been denying what's really going on in my family, including within my family of origin and my current family.	☐ True ☐ False
I am concerned about changes that will need to happen in my family for the cycle of obesity to be broken and for me, my child, and family to be well.	☐ True ☐ False

How did you go with answering the questions? Has it highlighted to you any areas where you make decisions that are perpetuating the cycle of negative behaviours in you, your child and family?

I know if you've been honest, there will be areas (as there are in all of us) where you'll need to develop a stronger 'no' muscle.

Reflecting on your answers, can you identify one priority area in which you feel the greatest difference can be made by saying 'no'? Before you challenge me and say that saying 'no' is so negative, let me state clearly: saying 'no' to one thing, means saying 'yes' to something else. In this case, your 'no' is a big resounding 'yes' to a healthier, happier future.

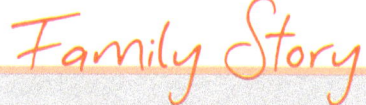

A mother learning to use her power of 'no'

One mother I have met recently had committed to her son's health and wellbeing, having decided it was no longer possible to take her son to community and family functions where there was an excess of unhealthy food that triggered her son's negative behaviour around food and sabotaged all her good work. As a consequence of her decision, she received negative criticism and unhelpful comments from family and her community. In fact, she was very much excluded from her community. However, despite that, she held firm to her why. Although this was not easy, her experience highlights the courage that is necessary to say 'no' and stick with it. If you asked her whether she would change her 'no' to 'yes', I know what she'd say, and I think you do too.

With this in mind, let's get serious. Identify one area that is important for saying 'no'.

Building your 'no' muscle

Now that you understand the importance of saying 'no', it's time to work out the priority areas where this muscle will start to be developed. Write your notes here so it's clear in your mind where this muscle is most important for you.

My priority area for saying 'no' is

This is my priority area because

What difference will it make to your life if you say 'no' in this area?

Now you've decided on your priority area for saying 'no', it's time to start building your 'no' muscle. I recommend focusing on this priority area for a specific time, say, at least a month, until you feel robust enough to say 'no' without guilt, shame or anxiety.

As Roslyn outlines in her book, which I highly recommend you read, there are many ways to become fluent in the 'language' of saying 'no'. She acknowledges that initially, it can be difficult to say 'no' when we've always said 'yes', but Ros reminds people the initial discomfort gradually shifts as we start to experience a different feeling – our improved self-worth. Here are her suggestions for building your 'no' muscle.

1. **Recognise how you feel when you say 'yes' when you really want to say 'no'.** Often this manifests as anxiety, resentment and guilt. When we say 'yes' and mean 'no', we're actually creating a conflict within bodies (and minds) and not being honest. We are not aligned with what we know is right for us. Wanting to say 'yes' is related to the very human desire for acceptance. For example, this is why we cave in when our friend asks us to coffee and cake, even though we know this is not a healthy decision for us at this time.

2. **Slow down your response to any requests (partners, kids, family and friends included).** Instead of agreeing to something immediately, allow yourself the time and space to consider if it's right for you. In our desire to please people, we often respond immediately and then feel resentful later. We even lie and make up stories to get out of what we agreed to, which in turn spirals us into more shame and guilt. By slowing down your response, you can determine if something is right for you or not. For someone committed to helping their family get well, any 'yes' must align with the goal of breaking the cycle of obesity. For example, if your child is persistently and inappropriately asking for food, you can respond by saying you will consider it, but not right now. Or you can refer to the menu plan you've already established and show your child when he or she is allowed treat foods.

3. **Prepare your response.** For example, knowing your child will ask for certain foods (based on past experience), it's critical you prepare responses so you're ready for that eventuality. Prepare what you might say at a family function when pressured into eating more food when you don't want to. While not foolproof, these preparatory responses will equip you and make it easier to respond with certainty and confidence in the face of the inevitable resistance you'll experience.

While this approach is extremely useful for dealing with your child, it is also an invaluable approach for managing any relationship, including with your partner, parents and extended family while navigating your health journey. Chances are they will also be resistant to change as your new behaviour shines a spotlight on their own entrenched ways of doing things.

Saying 'no' around food

When a child is demanding food, it can be very tempting to give in. Here's what you can do to exercise your 'no' muscle and hold firm to your commitment to a healthier life.

 ### Building your 'no' muscle

Take your priority area for saying 'no' and write down three things you can do to develop your 'no' muscle. For example, prepare a response for when your child demands food they don't need.

1.

2.

3.

You could also make a list of ten benefits to your child and to you from saying 'no'. This might sound like a lot, but when we see the benefits in black and white, our resolve strengthens. Here are a couple of examples to get you started.

- By saying 'no', I am being true to myself and putting the health of myself, my child and my family first.
- Making our health and wellbeing our highest priority gives us the best chance of overcoming the cycle of obesity in our family.
- When we do this, we become a good example to other people, perhaps giving them courage to take steps towards a healthier life.

You get the idea. Looking at things from this perspective, it's not hard to come up with ten benefits. Now it's your turn:

1.
2.
3.
4.
5.
6.
7.
8.
9.
10.

What happens when you can't say 'no'?

If you experience any level of anxiety around conflict, you may also find that the very idea of saying 'no' to a strong-willed person – yes even a child or teenager – can send you into a physical state of extreme anxiousness. This in turn leads to an easy back step on your attempts to set firm boundaries.

After you've become aware of the area in which you need to say 'no', when you say 'yes' instead, you may feel a physical and emotional response that is a clear indicator you haven't done what's best for you. The physical symptoms you may experience include the following:

- Sweating and increased heart rate.
- Headaches and butterflies in the stomach.
- Dizziness to the extent you might need to sit down.
- Nausea and vomiting.
- Extreme tiredness or heaviness, like you can't do anything and need to rest.

Emotions that arise might include:

- A feeling of anxiety and panic, or being overwhelmed.
- Depression, like you don't have control over the situation and feel like giving in.
- Hopelessness, like nothing you do makes a difference.
- Resentment about taking action that doesn't serve you.

These physical and emotional symptoms are an expression of being in a state of chronic stress. Studied in detail by my mentor, Professor George Chrousos, Chronic Stress Syndrome leads to excessive production of many hormones, including cortisol, that contribute to weight gain, fatigue and depression.[31]

Without becoming too technical, I feel it's important for every parent with a child living with obesity to become familiar with the boundaries that will make a positive difference to their child's life. Saying 'no' is not easy, but it is essential for a healthier life.

Saying 'no' is not a new parenting fad

After over 30 years of clinical practice as a children's doctor, I've observed how parenting has changed, a fact reflected most profoundly in parents' unwillingness to accept they will not always make their children happy with their decisions. As parents, our job is to raise resilient and healthy children. Saying 'yes' all the time denies them the opportunity to be fully human and experience that not everything will go their way. Said another way, there are times when a 'no' is entirely appropriate and healthy.

Developing resilience comes through life experiences that challenge us to grow. If children are constantly entertained and have their every need met at the moment it arises, they gain a distorted view of how life really is. A sense of entitlement learned as a young child can then lead to life becoming even harder when bigger challenges arise. From exams, friendships and even work issues, learning how to manage one's own expectations and those of other people you are required to engage with is a simple and important life skill.

It is better for your kids to know life is challenging, but also joyous and rewarding, and that though there are many mountains to climb the view from the top is always worth the effort of the climb. If parents continue to say 'yes', when a healthy 'no' is appropriate and essential for their children's good health and life, they are effectively condemning them to an existence in which they're unable to navigate any challenge. It's irresponsible and unfair to our kids.

Even though I love cycling stories, I often use the analogy of a surfboard rider in this context. When you're in the surf, you never know from which direction the next wave will come to knock you off the board. Being resilient requires you learn to cope with the unexpected 'waves of life'. Working on your 'no' muscle is an effective way to teach your children this vital life skill. In turn, they learn the value of saying 'no' too, and can start to apply it responsibly in their own lives. What a wonderful gift.

Resources

 Make sure you also get across to the Ride to Life website and access all the online resources that are available there.

In this stage, I've referred to Roslyn's book *Emotional Sobriety* on co-dependence. I highly recommend this as a resource for any parent wanting to establish and hold strong healthy boundaries for themselves and their child. Roslyn's website: www.roslynsaunders.com.au links you to Roslyn's helpful coaching support programs and the Power of 'No' Facebook group.

Dr John Rosemond, the parenting guru, provides useful tips on how to navigate this process effectively: www.parentguru.com

Triple P – Positive Parenting Program is a world evidenced-based program pioneered by Professor Matthew Sanders, an old colleague of mine at The University of Queensland: www.triplep-parenting.net.au/au-uken/triple-p

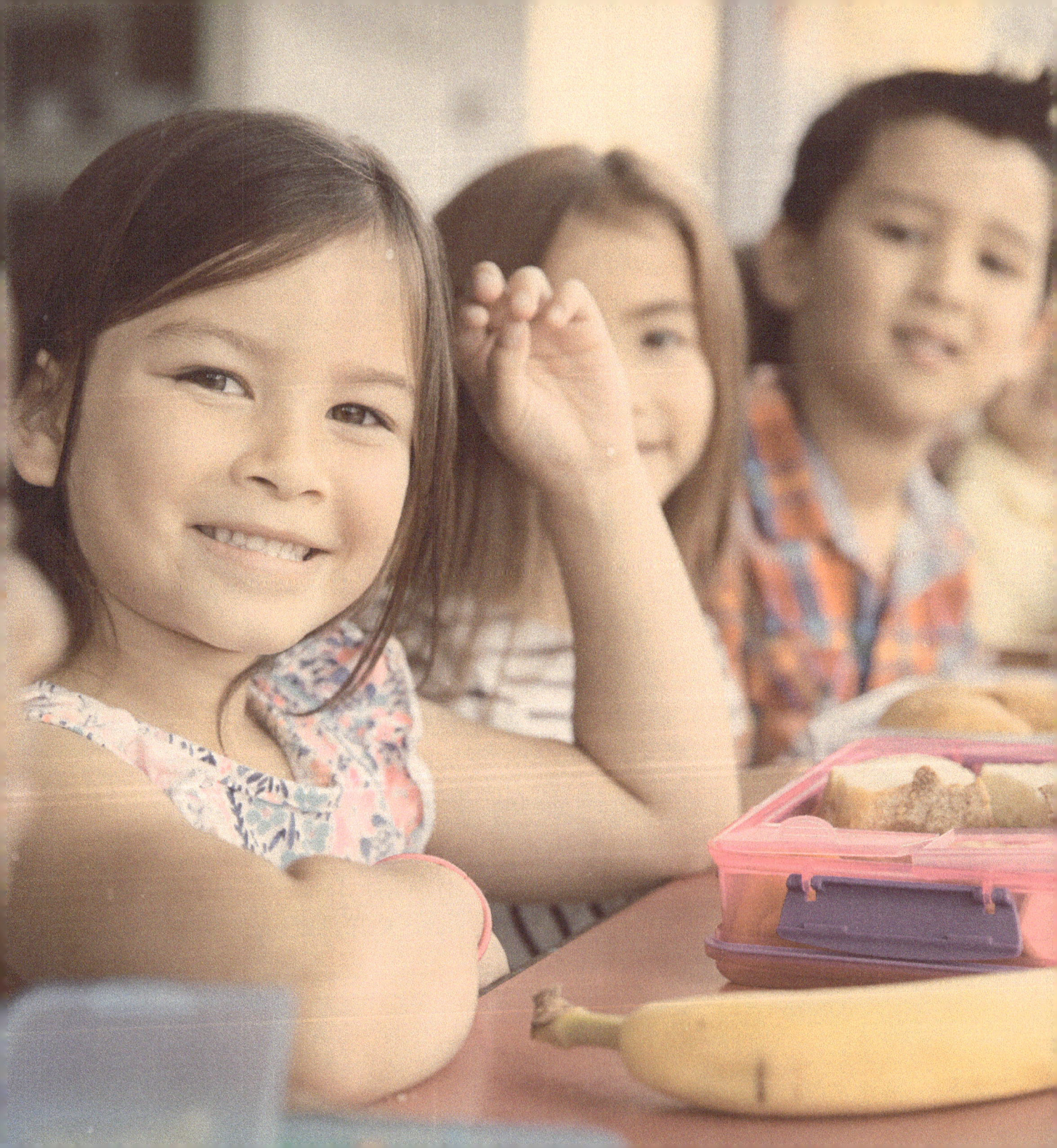

Stage 10

Body image, self-esteem and communication

> *To me, beauty is about being comfortable in your own skin. It's about knowing and accepting who you are.*
>
> Ellen Degeneres, TV Host, Comedian, Writer, (1958–)

In this stage, we will:

- Discuss the importance of having a positive body image.
- Look at strategies for building self-esteem.
- Outline how positive communication can improve family relationships and aid your child on their recovery.

Obesity is a very sensitive issue for many people, adult and child alike. Negative body image and low self-esteem can fuel the obesity cycle causing continued harm across the generations. Helping your child to navigate these concerns while simultaneously encouraging them to improve their habits can be tricky. On one hand, you are trying to help them to attain a healthier weight but on the other hand, you want to build their confidence and love for themselves at the same time. These two things can feel at odds with one another. In this stage we will discuss how to approach your child to help them feel encouraged, supported and loved, no matter what their weight.

Your influence as a parent

I've said several times that parents should never underestimate their own influence over their children. While this is true for eating and exercise habits, it's also true for body image and self-esteem. If your child has witnessed you expressing negativity toward your body, their body or others' bodies, they may internalise this message. For people struggling with obesity, shame and guilt about their bodies may be heavy and difficult emotions to conquer. Setting a good example of body positivity for your child is key to breaking the cycle of obesity. We are all made in different shapes and sizes. Your child is more than just their weight.

- Be mindful of how you talk about your body. Do you comment negatively about your weight or your body? Do you make comments about others' appearances? Do you make comments about specific parts of your body that you call 'fat' or 'ugly'? Do you compare your body with others?
- Keeping in mind that obesity is often an issue that occurs over generations, what kind of messages did you receive from your parents about appearances and weight? Do you recall kindness or criticism being levelled at those struggling with obesity? What kind of value did your parents place on appearances?
- Make a commitment to cease making negative comments about your, your child or others' bodies. Denigrating ourselves or others does not help anyone to address their health issues.

If you have personally struggled with body image, consider talking about your feelings with a professional. Contact your GP and speak to a counsellor or psychologist to help manage these negative feelings.

Talking about obesity with your child

While you are tackling a life-threatening challenge in helping your child recover from obesity, it is important to speak with care and sensitivity to them about the issue. Harassing them or bombarding them with constant criticism will only serve to worsen the situation. When you talk to the family about the changes you want to make to habits and routines, focus on *health*, not weight loss. Tackle the issue at a family level so that your child doesn't feel singularly targeted. When you are speaking to them specifically about their body, avoid using words like 'fat' or 'bad' or 'heavy'. Try not to use terms like 'the weight'. Refer to their weight as 'above a healthy range' rather than specifically calling them obese. Emphasise that we all come in different shapes and sizes and every one of us is special in some way. The journey you are on is to improve your health, not to drastically change your appearance.

Refer to obesity as a disease, a condition like other treatable illnesses. It is not inherent in the child. It is not a reflection of them as a person. Emphasise that it is definitely not a reflection of their value as a person.

Dealing with other family members

While you may seek to provide a nurturing, loving, kind environment for your child to embark on their recovery, other family members may cause harm and distress to your child with their comments or teasing. 'Funny' nicknames to do with appearance, 'light-hearted' barbs or 'helpful' comments from 'concerned' relatives that are really just an excuse to shame you and your child are unwelcome, unwarranted and unconstructive. It can be difficult to know how to respond to these behaviours. Certainly, you can attempt to ignore them, but if your child is being made miserable by misguided family members, you need to take them aside and ask them to desist from their behaviour.

Building self-esteem with your child

We all have value. Your child has many inherent, special and unique qualities, talents and skills. Look for ways to praise and encourage your child that aren't connected to their body or appearance. For example, you might praise them for the effort they put into an assignment at school, for the kindness they show others, or for their skills in drawing, singing or storytelling. Praise them for their good behaviour as a way of encouraging them to repeat it.

One of the strongest ways to build self-esteem with your child is to spend time with them doing an activity they enjoy. Your recovery from obesity will involve at times painful or confronting steps, but not every moment of the way need be focused on food, eating or exercise. Just as important is prioritising fostering a loving connection with your child. Just saying 'I love you' or 'I like being with you' builds your child's self-esteem and confidence.

Talking about food with your child

Changing your eating habits will involve some explanation to your child as to why you are no longer eating particular foods. Rather than labelling some foods 'bad', consider labelling them with the frequency with which they should be eaten. So take-away pizza is a 'sometimes' food, not every day, but on occasion perhaps once a month ideally! Of course you can make your own pizza dough in a much healthier way (therootcause.com.au/multi-purpose-dough/#more-3420). Likewise try to avoid explicitly labelling some food as 'good', rather you can talk about the ways in which the food makes your child healthy. For example you might talk about how fish is good for their brain power and carrots for seeing better and broccoli or cauliflower for stronger muscles!

Resources

Make sure you also get across to the Ride to Life website and access all the online resources that are available there.

For more on building self-esteem, check out these resources on www.raisingchildren.net.au

Big Life Journal (biglifejournal.com/): A marvellous journal, weekly blog, newsletter and podcast for improving self-esteem, anxiety and self-identity in children (4–10 years) and adolescents 11+ years. BLJ helps parents navigate this challenging but amazing journey with their children.

Action for happiness (www.actionforhappiness.org): A movement of people committed to building a happier and more caring society. A great resource that will help all the family, based on the principle that by helping others builds one's own happiness.

The Obesity Collective and Obesity Australia (www.obesityaustralia.org): The Collective is a platform for committed individuals and organisations from across the community to take on the obesity challenge together, with empathy and a whole of society perspective.

Notes

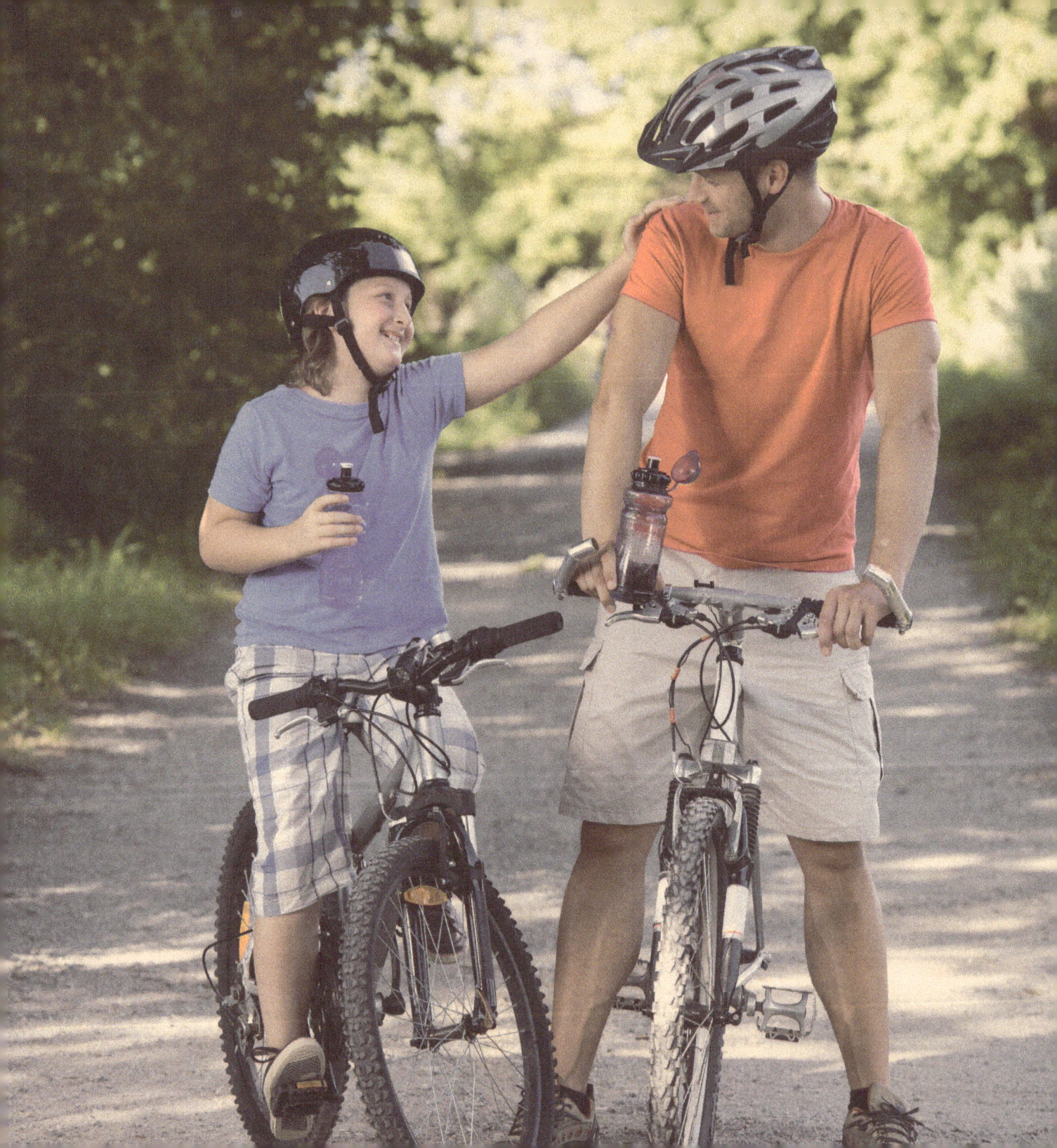

Stage 11

Setbacks and relapses:
why they happen and how to get back on the bike

It always seems impossible until it's done.

Nelson Mandela, the first black president of post-apartheid South Africa (1918–2013)

At this point in the book, I feel it's necessary to remind you that as a cyclist, I have had my shares of falls from my bike. In the worst case, after falling from my bike, I was unable to get up off the road. It was a serious accident, and it took surgery and six months of rehabilitation before I could get back to riding again. I felt disappointed, sad, frustrated and, at times, very depressed. The good news is I managed to get back up and riding again. And you can too, after any setback.

In this stage, we will:

- Cover strategies to help you and your family face the inevitable challenges of continuing your recovery.
- Remind you that having started your healthier journey to reclaim your child's life, healthy rewards along the way are important for maintaining momentum.

Learning and growing from experience

Setbacks will occur on your journey. They can be disappointing and leave you feeling dejected and ready to give up. If you do not allow yourself to feel that disappointment, but focus on what you can do better next time rather than focusing on the past action, which you cannot change, it will pass more quickly. Thereafter, the benefit of the setback will emerge through that fog to reset your compass towards your healthy goal.

When you have setbacks, avoid making it a reason to give up. Instead, take it as an opportunity to learn and reinvigorate your healthy journey. If we are open to it, the lesson from the experience will present itself. It follows that an essential step in this process is to allow the space and time for the lesson to integrate. Without allowing the time, it's very likely you will experience the same or worse setback within a short space of time. However, if you give yourself permission to acknowledge what has occurred, you can identify the triggers, situations, or people that led to the 'crash'.

Family Story

The food and mood connection

Brian and his sister Marjorie both attended my clinic together with their mother because of concerns about being obese and the strong family history of diabetes and heart disease on both sides of the family.

Brian had severe autism and several food intolerances while Marjorie had ADHD and anxiety. Both children were severely obese most of their childhood. At age nine years, Brian already weighed 55kg and by age 12-and-a-half his weight peaked at 87kg. Marjorie was at a similar weight at age 11 years and seven months.

Due to the challenging behaviours of both children, there was high intake of processed foods and carbohydrates. With maternal resolve, the family changed their nutrition enormously to a healthy high-protein, healthy-fat and low-carbohydrate nutritious diet with lots of fruits and vegetables, and less bread, pasta and rice.

This improved both children's behaviour as well as leading to significant weight loss as both children were less hungry when they had a good intake of eggs, fish and other healthy protein sources, and a larger intake of fibre in fresh fruit and vegetables.

Marjorie lost almost 14kg over the year while Brian lost about 8kg with major improvement in their BMI and waist circumference.

This amazingly inspiring mother and family showed the intimate connection between food, mood and behaviour.

Setbacks are common

Take small steps consistently

I've spoken previously about the beneficial gains to be made through effective and positive habits. New habits support you in breaking the cycle of obesity. They also keep you going when temptations to deviate from the journey show up. I reiterate the necessity of taking small steps consistently as this allows the integration of new behaviours which are setting you up for a healthier, happier life. Remember:

- Changes will take time.
- Be patient with yourself, your child and your family. They are learning too, and will also fall off the bike from time to time.

Nobody can be perfect all the time. Recognition and understanding of where they're at is essential, as is the maintenance of your own regular self-care regimen. By looking after yourself well – physically, mentally, emotionally – you give yourself the best chance of continuing to lead your family to a healthier, happier life. You also set a wonderful example to your family. And remember your support structure. Call upon these people to strengthen your resolve and go on.

Getting back on the bike after a setback

When you do experience a setback, there are some practical steps you can take to get back on track.

Identify your triggers or hooks

It is likely there will be a consistent theme to the trigger(s) that lead you (or your child) to 'fall' off the bike. Identifying the triggers will help you to put in place the necessary mechanisms by which you can prevent the trigger from setting you off in future.

A classic example mums relate to me is the drive home from after-school activities and work on a Friday night. At this time of the day and week, everyone is tired, often grumpy, and vulnerable. Invariably, one of the children demands takeaway food, and in response to his demands the mother finds it just so much easier to give in and drives into the closest fast-food drive-through. The child stops screaming, eats the food mindlessly, while the mother explodes and then spirals into guilt, shame and disappointment at having given in after being so resilient during the week.

Some practical ways this Friday night situation can be avoided include the following:

- Before you reach the point of giving in and blowing up, stop the car safely, take a deep breath, smile and relax (BSR – an old Buddhist practice). Continue breathing slowly and deeply until you feel calmer, allowing the repetitive hook and reaction cycle to be interrupted.
- In advance of driving home, plan the route so you avoid any visual triggers for the child caused by seeing familiar takeaway outlets.
- Ensure you have a healthy menu planned (and if possible ready to go) for Friday nights. This will happen if you've done your menu plan and shopped ahead. Having this prepared ahead of time will help.
- Have a healthy snack on hand to be eaten by the child if they're genuinely hungry.
- For a period of time, don't schedule activities on a Friday afternoon.

Applying the Just One Thing rule to triggers

Take a common trigger that causes you to respond in a negative way. Take your situation and plan a number of ways you can better manage it, considering your:

- Responses – are there things you could say differently? How could you respond differently, including not responding at all?
- Actions – is there more or less you could do in that situation? If so, what?
- Reflections – after the situation has passed, what learnings have you gained?
    1. One situation that triggers me is:
    2. I could handle this situation differently by:
    3. Things I could learn from past experience and apply from this point forward include:

Try working on this trigger for a period of time. Recognising it will take practice, as will interrupting the habitual negative response you've previously used in your chosen trigger situation.

It is likely it will take many times before you respond positively to this trigger. Be patient with yourself and, if you need to, talk with a trusted support person who can help you analyse your response and celebrate the wins when they happen.

Engage in mindful practices

As we touched on in stage 4, there are many paths to mindfulness, but they all have one common thread: they begin with the breath. A focus on your breath enables you to become centred and grounded, which means you're less likely to give in, be triggered, deviate from your goals and let your resolve dissolve.

Suggestions for bringing greater mindfulness around food and, indeed, all aspects of life include:

- Mindful breathing and meditation techniques
- Mindful movement, such as yoga
- Disconnecting from technology in all its forms for periods of time (even a short time can make a healthy difference)
- Journaling – for this I recommend having a look at Big Life Journal: www.biglifejournal.com
- Art therapy, and other alternative modalities, such as community choir singing
- Taking action to promote good mental health. One organisation doing good things in this arena is Action for Happiness. With their core mission being the promotion of mental health, they have wonderful resources for kids and adults: www.actionforhappiness.org.

I suggest researching these resources and then start with one technique that works for you. There are numerous benefits to be gained from mindful practices:

- Physiological benefits, such as a lowered heart rate and ability to respond to stressful situations in healthier ways.
- Reconnection with your body and senses.
- The ability to more sustainably manage the emotional aspects in the recovery from obesity.

You can teach your children these techniques, even doing them together – bonus connection value!

Meditation

Though I am not a Buddhist myself, I regularly practice Buddhist-style meditation, mindfulness, and Iyengar Yoga in order to reduce my stress, manage anxiety and assist with my physical wellbeing. As I place the highest value on my own health, I consciously and actively seek out these solutions to keep me healthy and happy.

I do not spend huge lengths of time meditating or undergoing meditative breathing exercises. In fact, most days I would only meditate for 15 minutes, but knowing it's important to keep it simple, I find these yoga-based breathing exercises very useful for my own health, and I highly recommend them to you and your family, including your children.

A meditation exercise

Begin practicing these exercises, even if initially for only a few minutes, together or alone at a regular, accessible time of the day.

- Find a quiet place or room to start.
- When ready, sit up straight in a comfortable chair with your legs slightly apart, relaxed with your hands either resting calmly on your thighs or clasped gently in your lap. Then close your eyes gently.
- Scan the different parts of your body starting from the top of your head, slowly moving down to your feet and toes. Focus on the different areas of your body and feel where you are tense or uncomfortable. Try to relax those areas of your body.
- Then observe your natural breath as you gently and slowly inhale and exhale through your nostrils. After a short time, usually a minute, you will begin to feel more relaxed and calm.
- Once you have reached this calmer state, with a steely focus, narrow your concentration to the sensation you experience as you breathe naturally, in and out through your nostrils.
- When you think you are ready – and your body will tell you when this occurs – start taking a deeper inhalation through your nostrils. At the end of your full inhale, gently pause for a moment at the peak before gently exhaling out through your nose as completely as you can.
- At the end of your exhalation, pause for a moment again before you begin the next cycle of deep slow inhalation and exhalation. Continue this for as long as you feel comfortable and enjoy the relaxing feeling coming over your body and mind.

I suggest practising regularly for three minutes initially and working up to ten minutes. If you practice every day at a regular time, you will soon reap the health benefits of this deep and consistent meditative breathing exercise. If after trying the technique outlined above you noticed some benefits, I encourage you to investigate breathing and meditation practices further. I am a firm believer in the mental, emotional and physical benefits of managing our emotions in breaking the cycle of obesity.

If meditation is something you feel is hard for you, then start with this as a beginning point. Simply sit still for a few minutes, breathing slowly in through your nose and out through your mouth, focusing on the air going all the way down to your stomach, not just to your chest. Think about the air as it goes into your body, slowly circulating through it, and then slowly being released again. You can do this with your eyes either closed or open but looking at something simple like waves, raindrops, candle flame, a colour pattern. Sometimes this can be just as effective as a means of slowing down your breathing, and shifting your energy and attention from one thing to another. It's also a great stress management technique. As you get good at this, try extending it for longer, and then tackle the exercise noted above using just your nose for inhaling and exhaling.

Resources

Make sure you also get across to the Ride to Life website and access all the online resources that are available there.

Meditation phone apps for kids and adults:

Dr Koala recommends the following apps:

Free apps (or an added small cost):
- Smiling Mind
- Insight Timer
- Headspace Meditation & Sleep
- Calm

Paid apps
- Buddhify: Dr K uses this one – very adaptable to your life!
- Wild Journey: mindfulness meditation within nature

For deeper meditation discussion about the benefits and science of meditation explore the following.

B. Alan Wallace, a pioneer in studying the interface between Tibetan Buddhist meditation and Western Science and Philosophy: www.alanwallace.org/

Tanzin Palmo, English Tibetan Buddhist nun whose biography *Cave in the Snow: Tenzin Palmo's Quest for Enlightenment* in 1998 describes her 12 years in solitary retreat in a cave in the Himalayas. She is one of Dr Koala's most inspiring people he has the pleasure to meet and hear talk.

Pema Chodron, an American Tibetan Buddhist nun: pemachodronfoundation.org/. Another amazing Buddhist nun with wonderful teachings to address the power of kindness to address the world's suffering.

Notes

Notes

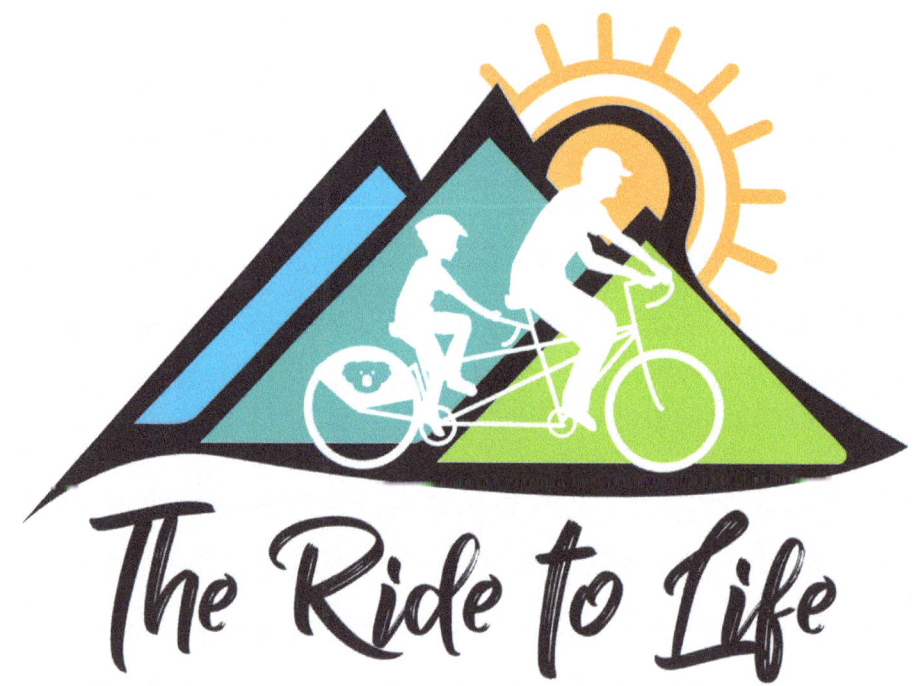

PARTIE 4
MAINTAIN AND SUSTAIN
Staying on the bike even after the main event

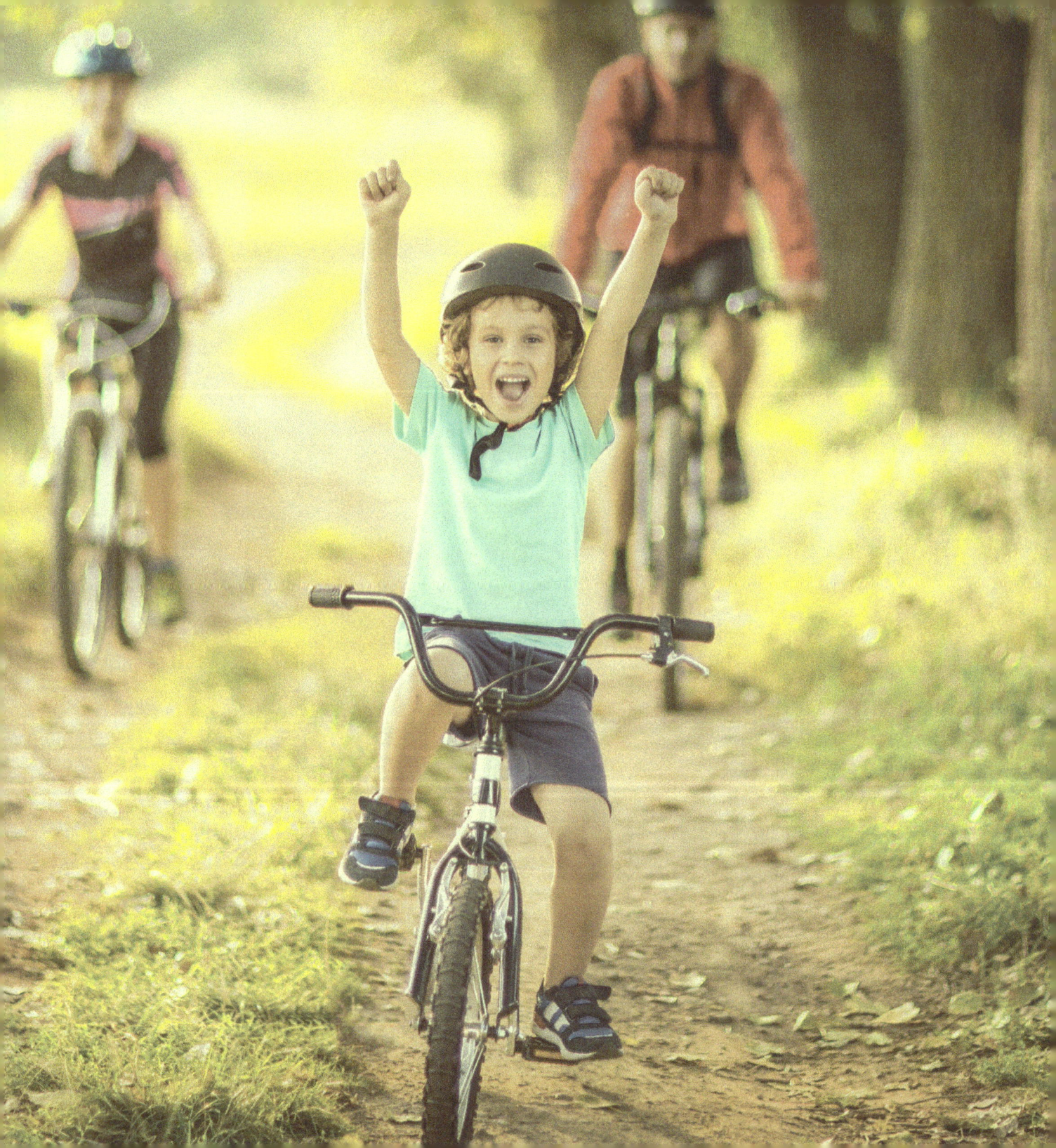

Stage 12

The future's bright: dreaming big and creating a new reality

> What you can do or dream you can, begin it.
> Boldness has genius, power, and magic in it.
>
> *Johann Wolfgang von Goethe, German writer and poet (1749–1832)*

It can be very easy to get bogged down in everyday life. When problems become overwhelming and it's hard to see beyond the day, let alone the week, we lose sight of the fact that there is more to life than our problems.

We live in a world where it can feel like external influences, such as our social peers (the 'Joneses'), media (especially social media), celebrities and global challenges (for example, terrorism, climate change, the obesity epidemic and addiction in all its forms), dictate our lives. It's human nature to be concerned; however, these influences distract and take us away from ourselves and what's really important for us and our family to be healthy and happy. Focusing externally, we lose sight of our own core values and the compass that directs us to the best (and healthiest) pathway for us.

In this stage, we will:

- Explore the idea that there's value in having a dream (or two) for you, your child and your family.
- Present the idea of the field of possibilities and how you can integrate this into your life in small ways.
- Start the process of imagining a more fulfilling and purposeful life for you and your family.

Everybody's got a dream, even if it's buried a little deeper than we'd like

By looking inward, we can reflect on the things that are important to us. Internal reflection is important for the following reasons:

- Without this reflection you don't have clarity about where you are now and where you'd like to go.
- Everybody needs a dream to inspire and give them hope and purpose.
- By having a dream, no matter how big or small, and pursuing it, you become a leader within your own family, setting an example for your children and all in your family to follow. What an inspiration!

I want to remind you not to underestimate the power you have to inspire your children and become the most important role model in their lives. I also want to remind you of my earlier statement around external role models. I see many parents looking to other people to be the important influences in their children's lives. While others do have a role, by comparison to the influence you can have, just because you're present every day in their lives, you have the potential to be the strongest and most effective and important role model for them.

By now you will understand this book is about you gaining healthy control over your life and your family. Working through each of the areas we've covered in the book and slowly integrating the various positive changes, you will notice space open up in your mind, allowing you to consider possibilities you hadn't envisaged previously.

This is the time to start dreaming about how you would love your life to be. To be clear, I am not talking celebrity lifestyles or winning the lottery. Instead, I am talking about keeping it real and being honest by identifying what makes sense for you. For some it might be planning and taking their first family holiday at the beach. Others may be inspired to participate in a family challenge together, such as a five km family fun run or walk for charity; learning to ride a bike or skateboard, play the piano, win a writing competition or spelling bee, or making a new friend – all these are things we might dream about. Take action towards making your dream a reality – those first steps are powerful ways to affirm a dream and turn it into a goal.

It really doesn't matter what your inspiration is; it's just important that you find something to work towards. For me, joining the Smiling for Smiddy cancer charity allowed me to cycle around the world and make amazing new friends. More importantly, it allowed me to raise important research funds to help young people suffering from different cancers, such as melanoma. Although being part of a 'tribe' like Smiling for Smiddy inspired me, it's my hope that my actions have inspired my family and other people to live healthier lives.

There are many ways you can go about creating your dream and I'm offering just one way here. When I'm dreaming big, I find it helpful to create mind maps. A mind map is a tool for capturing your ideas, thoughts and images within a single diagram. A visual thinking tool, it will help to structure your ideas and identify what's most important in pursuit of your dream.

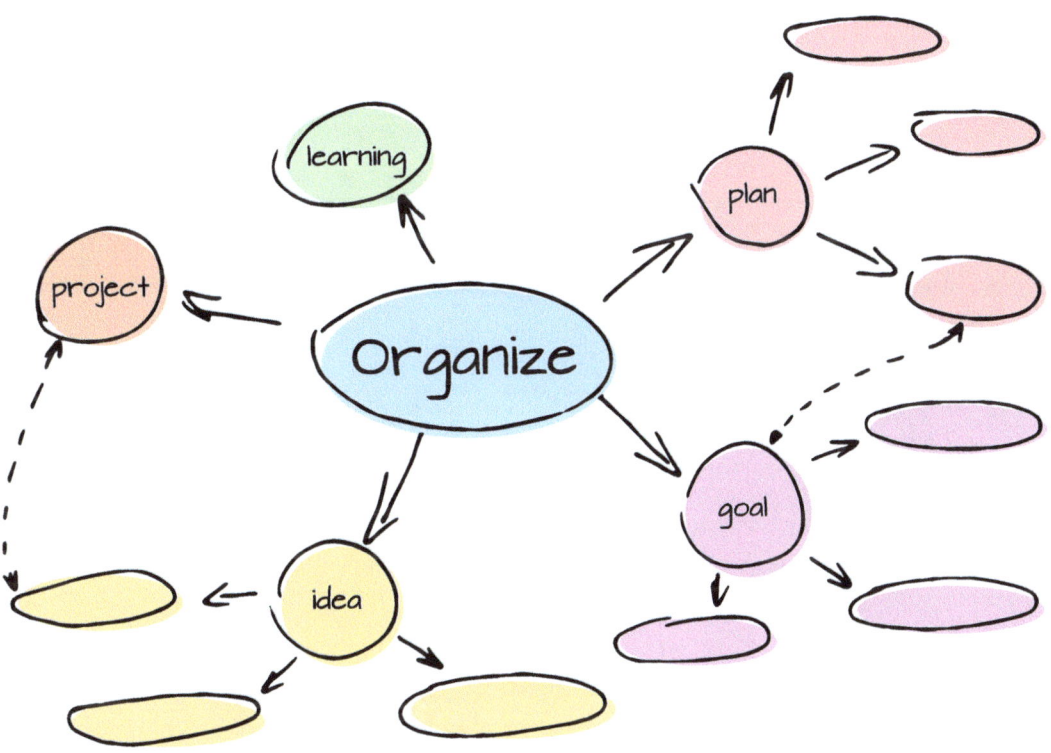

This exercise is about letting your imagination run free

To do this requires you let go of all your preconceived ideas about what is possible in your life. We each have our own limitations. These can be physical, financial, personal, social and so on, but this exercise is about considering what you would love to do, if the limitations didn't exist. You may choose to complete this exercise on your own or with a trusted friend or support person from your network.

For this exercise, you will need:
1. Blank sheets of paper
2. Some colouring pencils or pens
3. Quiet time and place
4. A support person (optional).

The steps for creating a mind map are as follows:
1. Choose a central idea. The central idea is the starting point of your mind map and is what you're exploring. Place the central idea in the middle of the page.
2. Add 'branches' to your map, using different coloured pencils. There is no limit to the number of branches, but start with four.
3. Add some key words to the map, working on the principle of one key word per branch. Each word then stimulates thinking around other associated ideas. Document these in the mind map, using the different colours to 'code' the ideas.
4. Include images/drawings in the mind map. You don't need to be an artist. Drawings can be simple and are there for the purpose of visually representing your idea.[32] Focus on the feelings you'll have as you work towards, and then see, your dreams come to life.

There are also online mind mapping apps, however, I feel that putting pen to paper is just as good, if not better than any digital version of your mind map. The value of the mind map is that it stimulates creative thinking, which may have been dormant for some time. I encourage you to approach this exercise with an open mind in the knowledge that if you're able to create your first mind map, you now have the skills for thinking creatively about other aspects of your life.

Obviously, there is no magic wand that will bring your dream to life immediately; however, without this fundamental step of thinking creatively about what you'd love life to look like, it will be difficult to imagine a healthier and happier one beyond the current challenges.

Moving forward

Reflecting on the mind map, is there one thing you can do to begin the journey towards fulfilling your dream? For example, if your dream is to complete a charity fun run/walk as a family, can you make a time to share your dream with your family. Whether your family come on board immediately or not, it's vital *you* stick to your dream and start working through the steps to reach it. Your commitment and resolve to achieve your dream are what counts. Keep going regardless. As you move towards your dream, support *will* come from surprising avenues, perhaps even from the initially uncommitted family members!

As you become more confident with mind mapping, you may wish to use this tool with your child, helping them to create a vision or dream for themselves. Keeping them focused forward on something other than their current challenges, this skill of learning to set and pursue an inspiring goal is an invaluable tool for life.

Try not to limit your goals and dreams to just eating healthily and being more active, although these goals are very important. It's as important to have dreams that reflect the other dimensions of life. People have always been inspired by nature, music and dance, art and literature and perhaps these things inspire you too. Look beyond your usual sources of inspiration to find things that really get your creative juices flowing.

Resources

Make sure you also get across to the Ride to Life website and access all the online resources that are available there.

I love the *Little People, Big Dreams* books for children by Isabel Sánchez Vergara , a Spanish author from Barcelona, Spain. Isabel has written about many famous artists, writers, musicians and inspiring world leaders in her children's books. My favourites are David Bowie, Steven Hawking and Marie Curie. We were all children once with big dreams! Some of us get to realise them, many more should! Follow her on instagram #mariaisabelsanchezvegara.

Also please use the growth mind set resources, including journals, blog and podcast from The Big Life Journal team for children and for teens, and parents and their teachers: biglifejournal.com

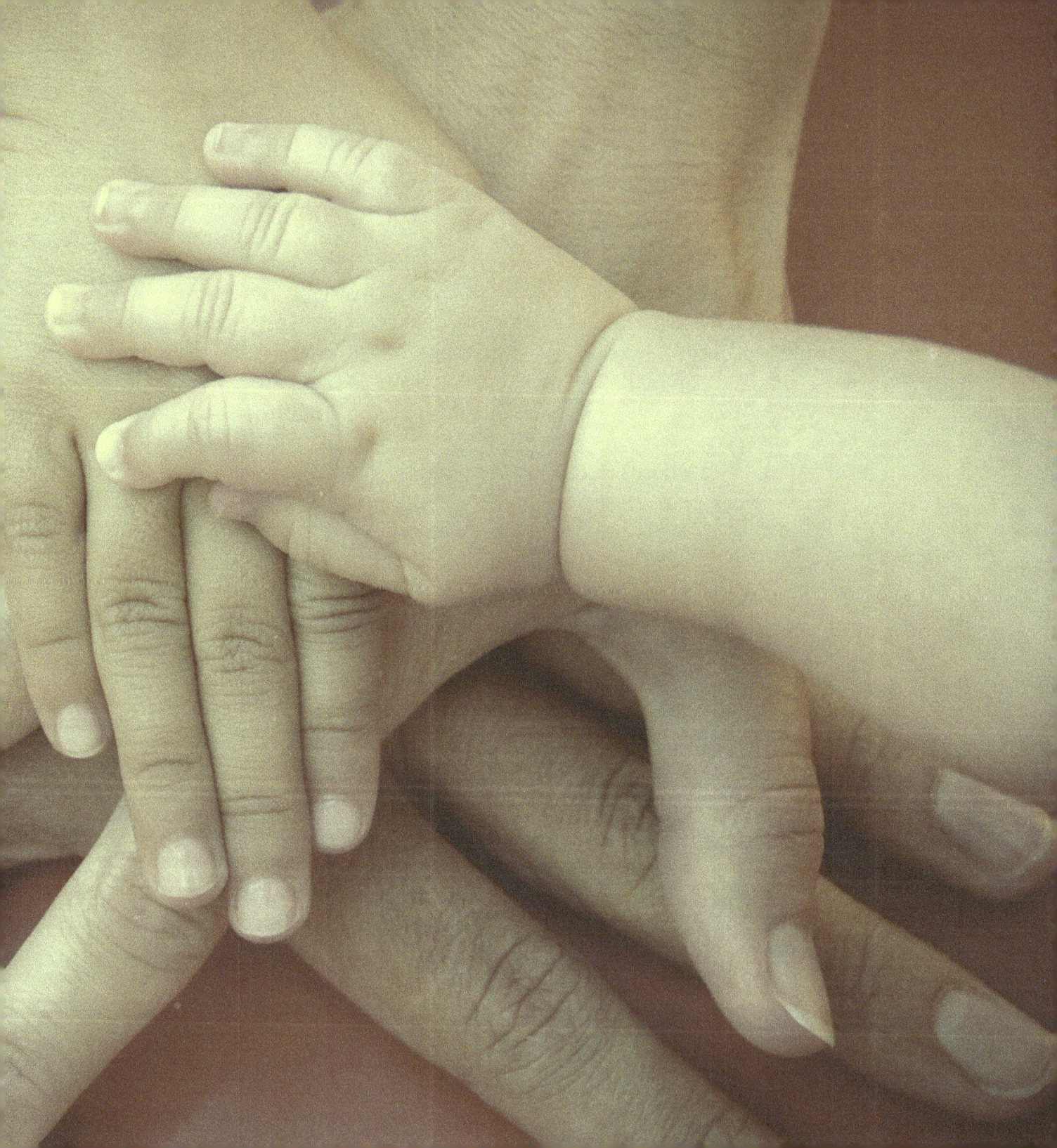

Stage 13

Connect and care: why community helps and how it pays to be part of one

> *In every community, there is work to be done. In every nation, there are wounds to heal. In every heart, there is the power to do it.*
>
> Marianne Williamson, American writer (1952–)

Studies have shown obesity can have an isolating effect on people.[33] Based on my own clinical experience, I can support these studies with anecdotal evidence. A common concern expressed by parents and patients in my clinic is that they feel alone as a result of their obesity. This experience is also evident in children and adolescents who become stigmatised, isolated and disconnected from social networks.

In this stage, we will:

- Discuss the importance of community on the journey to a healthier, happier life for you and your family.
- Consider the options for you when looking for community connections.

You're not alone

Examples of isolation among children living with obesity are all too familiar: an adolescent girl or boy with severe obesity is embarrassed by their body size and shape. Over time, this can lead to avoidance of social situations where their physical appearance would be observed (and potentially judged) by others, such as the beach, swimming pool or sporting activity.

Isolation can come in other ways too. The social stigma associated with obesity infiltrates many areas of life, including through professional channels. I've heard many stories from parents who have felt judged by the doctor or other health professional from whom they've sought advice and help.

Parents, teachers and friends can inadvertently or insensitively pass judgement on your situation, which is unhelpful and can be hurtful. Negative interactions like these perpetuate the feelings of guilt and shame in the parent, further isolating the family. While it's understandable to feel overwhelmed by these kinds of experiences, it is important you look beyond them and focus on your '**Why**' and where you're going.

I've already talked about developing your support network and community, in its many forms. These can provide valuable connections for you and your family as you work towards your goals and a healthier, happier life.

A study[34] that followed 60,000 Germans over 25 years found that happiness has more to do with our personal choices than it has to do with our genetic make-up and physical circumstances. The study found that helping others was more important than acquiring money. Another finding indicated that focusing on family, social activities, exercise, a spiritual practice and doing a healthy amount of service for others were good choices to ensure happiness.

How is this relevant to breaking the cycle of obesity in your family?

It's relevant because the better your connection to a community, the more likely you are to feel a sense of belonging. We are all social beings to some extent and need the connection that comes from being around like-minded people who support us and whom we can also support and encourage.

As I've noted previously, there is always someone in the world who is worse off than we find ourselves. By connecting with others in a community or 'tribe', you can identify others who are in similar situations and could benefit from your own learnings and experience. Helping others in this way is just another tool for keeping you on track to a healthier, happier life.

Looking for healthy community connections

If we've been disconnected from community for a long time, it may be difficult to know where to start. There is also the challenge of breaking into new groups, which can feel a little daunting. It's why I suggest to people to do a community scan first.

What do I mean by this?
- Look for organisations that are proven to focus on family and/or children's wellbeing. These may be organisations that have been around for many years, but could also include some that have been more recently established, such as online support groups. See the following page for a list of options.
- Source a balance of offline and online communities. While online communities have numerous benefits, such as providing much needed access to support for people in remote locations and connections with people globally, they should not be the only form of community support you seek.

When researching suitable communities, consider your needs, values and interests, and those of your child and family. Answer the following questions:
- What kind of community or organisation do you want to be part of?
- What would help you and your child to feel more connected?
- What activities would help promote your child's confidence?
- Is the community group aligned to your values and your goal/s?
- Do you have a sense of their approach to support? Are they encouraging and non-judgmental?
- Consider the cost of involvement from a financial and time perspective.

There may be some experimentation required before you find an exact match to your needs; however, this can be an enjoyable experience too. Many groups and organisations have a trial period that allows people to try the activity before they commit to it for a longer period. Be sure to take advantage of this opportunity if it's available.

Some examples of groups and organisations

- Cycling Australia and related state and territory cycling organisations: Bicycle NSW, Bicycle QLD, Bicycle SA, Bicycle Network Victoria and Tasmania, West Cycle (WA)
- The YMCA operate in all states of Australia
- Scouts Australia
- Girl Guides
- Sea Scouts
- PCYC
- Swimming Australia
- Surfing Australia
- Surf Life Saving Clubs Australia – Nippers
- Basketball Australia
- Netball Australia
- Soccer Australia
- Rugby Australia
- AFL Little League Australia
- Baseball
- Little Athletics
- Parks Australia
- Australian Marine Conservation Society
- Australian Geographic
- National Geographic
- Scuba Diving clubs
- World Wildlife Fund
- Australian Conservation Foundation
- Martial arts such as Tae Kwan Do or Karate

The benefits of being part of a community

There are many tangible benefits from being part of a community. We're more active; we make friends; we provide service; we connect. However, many of the benefits of community connection are unseen. They are discovered in the way they make us feel. Through increased physical activity, we feel better about ourselves and enjoy improved feelings of self-worth.

Through new friendships, we feel valued, appreciated and connected. We also feel joy and have fun. For many people these are experiences that have been absent from their lives for a long time. By giving service to others in healthy ways, we feel the all-important connection with others that make being a compassionate human being so special and unique.

Resources

A great place to start when seeking out community connections is to refer to your local council website. Often a great repository of information about organisations and events, your local council can point you in the right direction. I recommend starting there and then being open to where it can take you.

Make sure you also get across to the Ride to Life website and access all the online resources that are available there.

Notes

....

....

....

....

....

....

....

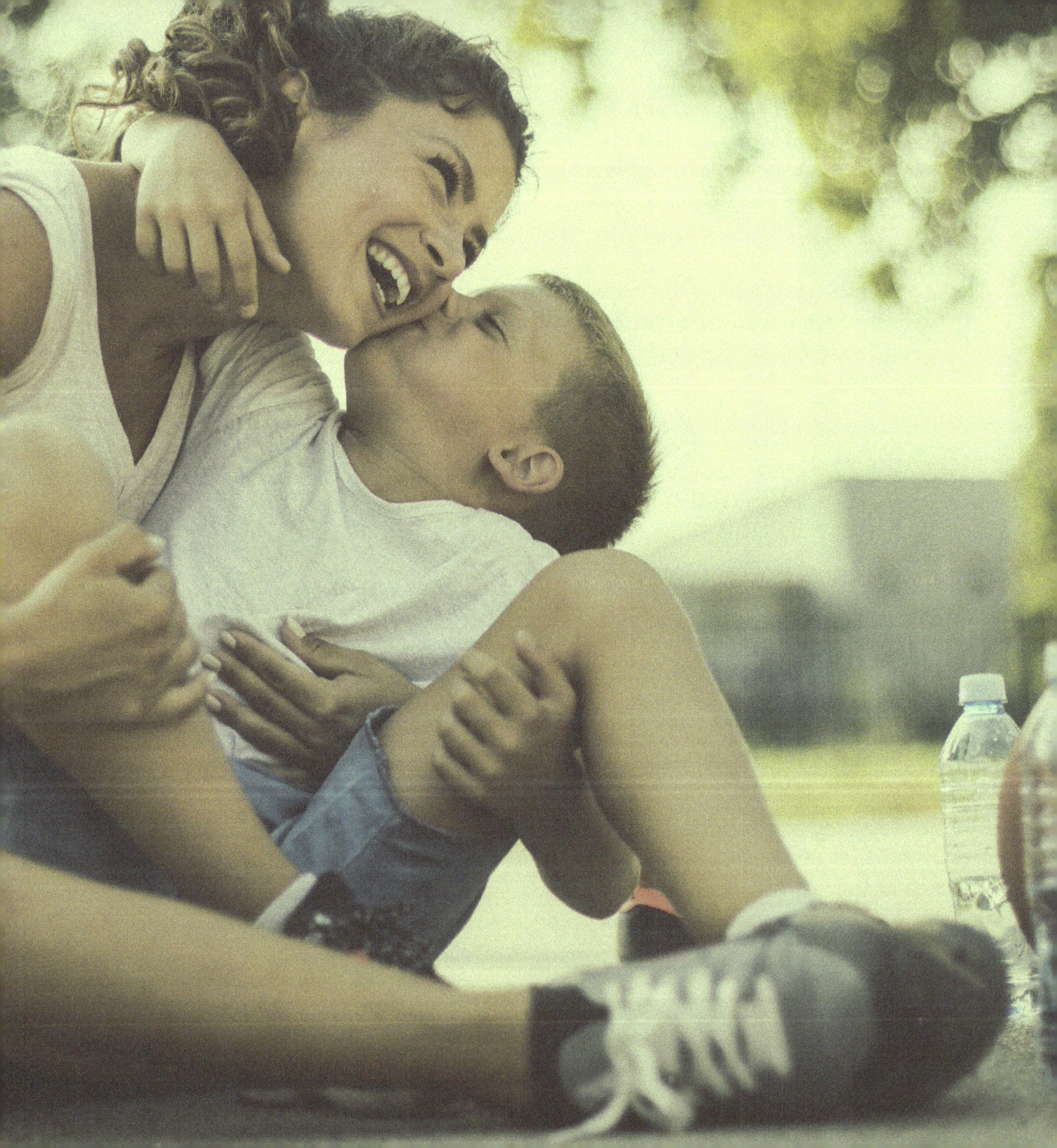

Stage 14

The final stage on your Champs-Élysées!

But don't forget Le Tour de France is on every year! So is your Ride to Life!
Well done, you! Regardless of whether you've read the book from start to finish, or have absorbed one stage at a time, completing each activity along the way, you are to be commended for reaching this point.

The consistent thread throughout this book is the focus on starting within and working outwards. Doing that requires patience and persistence, with ourselves and with our children. For us to bring about the change in health and wellbeing in our children, it actually starts with us. As we work to develop a healthier mindset and habits, the ripple effect occurs in our children with less effort than we'd expect. Just remember Charlie's Mum's inspiring story!

Breaking the inter-generational cycle of obesity is one of the most significant challenges humanity faces today. Coming from a medical background, I am grateful that research is being done to understand more about this chronic disease. It is a vital and essential component of piecing together the puzzle of obesity.

Equally as important, if not more so, is the work each individual must do in the process of recovery and healing from obesity and its many complications. In this sense, it is in our hands. It is the individual – faced with the condition – who must make healthier, wiser choices, based on their mental and emotional wellbeing. If parents and carers do not start making and demonstrating these wiser choices for their children, I feel there will be more challenging times ahead of us.

My own research in this area, coupled with my clinical work and my care of many families and their children with obesity has taught me that no amount of medical intervention can replace the conviction of a parent who is committed to saving and reclaiming good health for their child. Countless times I have seen parents, in the face of incredible challenge, rise up and take the steps towards a healthier life – both for them and their children. This takes enormous courage and honesty, particularly as it causes these parents to reflect deeply on their own lives and choices, and their own experiences during childhood, many of which are deeply buried. While too painful to face until now, these experiences still influence the way we act as a parent to our child.

While this book is a guide, I encourage you to think of it more as a companion. Providing reassurance and encouragement that you are on the right track, *Ride to Life* is a reminder that small steps taken consistently in the right places will yield the results you are striving for. I also encourage you to take advantage of the many resources that are available on the Ride to Life website. Transformational work like this cannot be done alone and parents, carers and children will benefit greatly from the Ride to Life community support.

Let's keep working together to break this devastating cycle of obesity and create a future filled with meaning, hope and purpose for our children and for ourselves. They, like us, deserve it. I truly hope you have gained strength and resolve through starting the Ride to Life program and have made the important mental shift towards creating a healthier, happier and more purposeful life for you and your children.

Dr Gary 'Koala' Leong

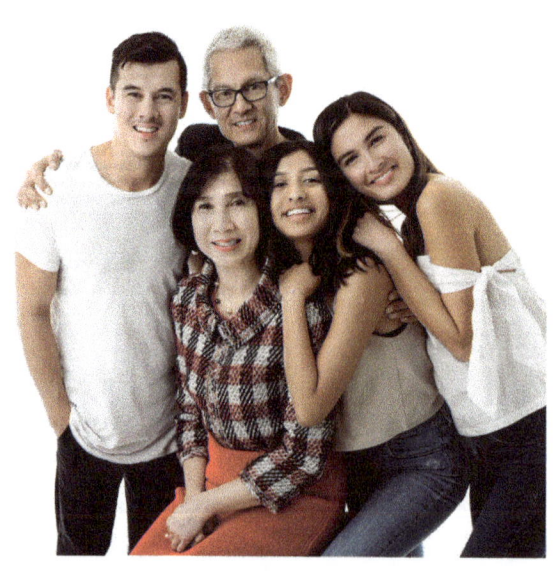

Acknowledgements

While my name appears on the cover of Ride to Life, pulling it together has involved the efforts of many, and it's here I'd like to acknowledge those many people in my lucky life.

First and foremost, I extend my sincerest gratitude and appreciation to my past and present patients. I have referred to them many times throughout the book and it is no understatement to say they have been my teacher. Only through them did I come to understand my purpose and desire to communicate the important messages in Ride to Life.

To Roslyn Saunders, a patient and loyal friend, whose persistent encouragement finally paid off and found me putting 'pen to paper'. Apart from your friendship, I truly value your wisdom and understanding of the connection between emotions and addictions. It has been a wonderful guide for me on my own healing journey.

Pulling the book together has been possible through the work of my first editor, Macushla Collins. I'm so appreciative of your capacity for understanding the deeper purpose behind my vision and I thoroughly enjoyed working together with you. I can highly recommend Macushla to budding authors who want to get their vision onto the page through utilising her own book *7 Day Book Blueprint: a step-by-step guide to planning, organising and writing a book when you don't know where to start*.

A special thanks to Ann Wilson, Dixie Maria Carlton and Samantha Sainsbury and Annette Welsford, for the assistance provided by you and your team through the publishing process. It has been wonderful to see the 'hard copy' come to life through your collective efforts. You got me going again when I had hit a wall – my Black Dog!

To the past and present research and clinical teams I've worked with, thank you for your enduring and collegiate support. Special thanks to my previous NIH mentors Professor Jim Segars and Professor George Chrousos and my PhD supervisors Professor John Eisman and Dr Edith Gardiner. Together, we're doing good work and through publications such as this, I am hopeful that long may it continue. A special thank you to all my clinical team at the Nepean Hospital within the Family Metabolic Health and Diabetes services; you are all very special and your dedication to help so many families with obesity and diabetes is amazing.

A special thanks to my great friend, cycling buddy and mentor Professor George Muscat, who has recently retired after an emeritus academic research career in metabolism and obesity research at the highest level. Now George all we have to do together is ride our bikes up and over those many beautiful mountains of the world that await us in many new adventures.

Also to all my Smiling for Smiddy family who have taught me really what is probably the most important thing in this crazy world, and that is to help others through service and philanthropy in this case for people with cancer and other health problems, including mental illness. It brings you both happiness and amazing friendships. A special mention of thanks and love to the SFS founder Mark 'Sharky' Smoothy and his darling wife Alyssa, Christian, Krista, Professor Glenn the Spiderman, Stinky Dave, Captain Davo, my fellow lantern rouge buddies in the SFS peloton who always encourage me to keep going, Damo, Ken and Ben, Wendy, Kevvies no 1 and no 2, Mia, Sammi-Jo, Felicity and Steve, Brooke and Serge, my Madrid to Lisbon hero Jim, Lesa, Julie, my pinot mates Nat, Phillip and Brett my doppelgänger, 'Sir' Michael the Lensbach, my amazing Brisbane to Townsville buddy Bruce and his beautiful wife Jenny, Kirsteen and John, my Big Brother Jeff, Andrew C., and so many more SFS friends!

A special mention to one SFS legend and friend 'Big Kev' Kevin Moultrie the founder of the Fab to be Fit Foundation www.fabtobefit.org.au and director of Transform-US-Fitness Kids www.transform-usfitnessforkids.com.au/. Big Kev's vision and passion for promoting children's health and fitness, life purpose and leadership though his unique school fitness programs is truely world-breaking. I am so proud to be part of the Fab to be Fit Foundation and I look forward with him to inspire so many more families and communities to be healthier, fitter and happier.

To my amazing five brothers and sisters-in-laws, my nephews and nieces and and my extended Leong-Lim family and my friends all over the world.

Namaste to all my wonderful Iyengar yoga teachers over the last 20 years that have nurtured and encouraged me to keep in the moment of the breath and pose, including Suzi, Robyn, Peta, Helen and Caroline and more recently Tamar and Henryk.

To my children, Martin, Julia and Vivienne, I love and appreciate your acceptance of me and my learning. Thank you for all you've taught me.

Finally, my sincerest thanks and love go to my beautiful and forever patient wife, Micky. Thank you for holding the space for me to pursue, and fulfil, my purpose. I am so grateful and love you for it.

About Dr Gary Leong

Dr Gary Leong is a paediatric endocrinologist who specialises in treatment of children suffering with obesity and diabetes and its complications. A humane and very real person – not just a medical doctor and PhD – Gary loves working with kids and their families to help them work towards enjoying healthier and happier lives.

For the people who care about letters and places, Gary's professional qualifications are substantial. He is an Associate Professor of Paediatrics at the University of Sydney Nepean Clinical School and Nepean Charles Perkins Research Hub in Western Sydney. He is a Senior Staff Specialist in Paediatric Endocrinology and Diabetes and the Clinical Paediatric Lead in the Nepean Family Metabolic Health Service and the Paediatric Diabetes Service at the Nepean Hospital. He is also in private practice at The Children's Clinic in Bondi Junction in Sydney.

For 12 years prior to this, Dr Leong maintained a joint clinical and research appointment at the Mater Children's Hospital and Queensland Children's Hospital (formerly Lady Cilento Children's Hospital) in Brisbane and The University of Queensland's Institute for Molecular Biosciences, where he conducted clinical and basic research into child obesity and metabolism.

He obtained a PhD from the Garvan Institute, The University of New South Wales in 2002 after completing his general paediatric and paediatric endocrine training in Sydney and around Australia in 1992. His medical degree was obtained from The University of Melbourne in 1982. Dr Leong has memberships of several national and international paediatric endocrine and research societies and was formerly the Chair of the Australasian Paediatric Endocrine Group Growth Hormone Advisory Committee, which assisted the Federal Department of Health by providing expert advice on growth hormone therapy in children with growth problems.

While Gary's research has taken him across the globe, from Sydney, Australia to the National Institutes of Health in Bethesda, Maryland, USA, it is his clinical work with children and their families that stimulated his desire to find practical ways to help families break the cycle of obesity.

As a witness to the devastation wrought by obesity on families, parents and children, Gary felt compelled to find simple and practical ways for them to reclaim their lives through sustainable changes that anyone can do, with the right mindset, habits and support. Integrating his personal love of cycling and long, challenging rides like Le Tour de France, Gary encourages the reader to get on their bike and stay on it, because the lives of their children depends on it.

Gary rides every year for various charities, but has been a great supporter of the Smiling for Smiddy Cancer charity which supports cancer research in melanoma at the Mater Foundation. More recently he has become a board member of the Fab to Fit Foundation which promotes healthy physical activity programs for children from socially disadvantaged communities where childhood obesity is highly prevalent.

Gary is a husband to Micky and proud father to three grown-up children. He has a large loving family who migrated here from Hong Kong in the mid 1960s when Gary was only 4 years old. He is a mad-keen cyclist and loves combining cycling with his great loves of travel and connecting with people, especially his family and the natural world.

Speaking opportunities

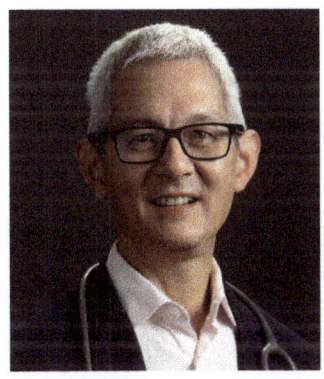

In addition to high demands on his professional knowledge and skills, Dr Gary Leong is a sought-after speaker for conferences and events. His key message for professionals and patients is consistent: healing and recovery from obesity is the responsibility of the individual, but nobody does it alone. It requires a team effort between parents and carers, children, and the medical and auxiliary professionals who are part of the journey towards a healthier and happier life.

Popular topics Gary speaks on include:

- The role of parents in a child's recovery from obesity and diabetes
- How medical professionals can facilitate a child's recovery from obesity and diabetes
- How parents and carers can navigate the recovery journey without losing their mind
- Practical steps to recovery for parents, children and professionals
- Why addressing obesity and diabetes is important for the health of the planet.

For more information, bookings or bulk book sales: childhoodobesityprevention.com.au

Image courtesy of Mark Marchand Lumapixel Studios, Sydney.

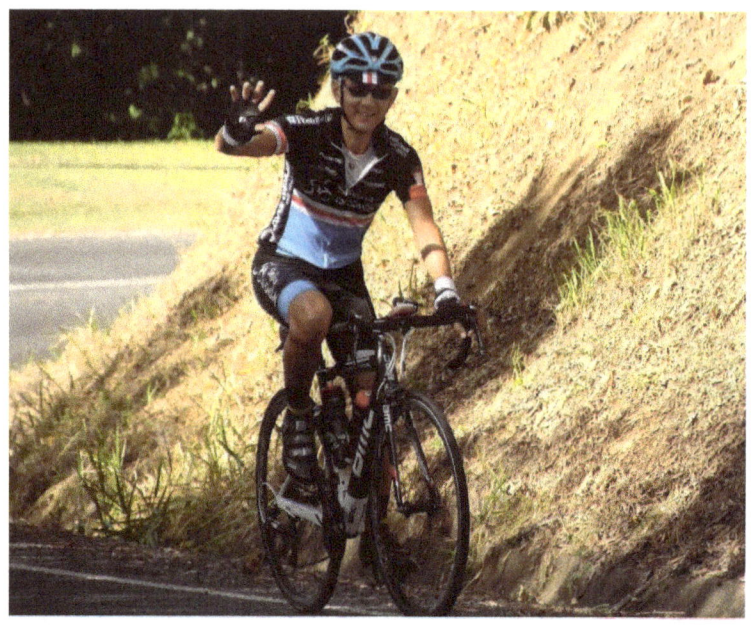

Dr Koala riding at 2016 Noosa Smiddy.
Image courtesy of Denise Barnett and the Mater Foundation.

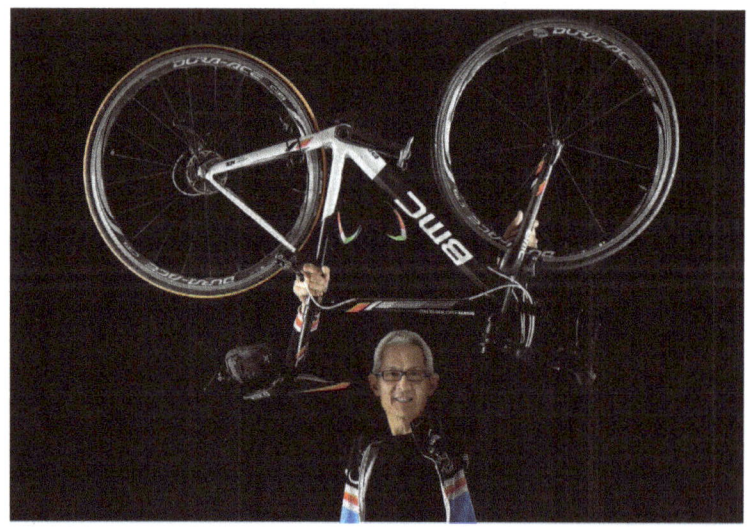

Dr Koala holding his Body-Mind Connection (BMC) machine which he rode for 1600km in 8 days from Brisbane to Townsville with 49 other Smiling for Smiddy heroes in the 2016 Smiddy Challenge.
Image courtesy of Gap studios, Sydney.

Endnotes

1. The GBD 2015 Obesity Collaborators, Health Effects of Overweight and Obesity in 195 Countries over 25 Years, July 6, 2017, Vol. 377, No. 1, pp. 13-27.
2. Melissa Sweet, The BIG fat conspiracy, ABC Books, 2007, p. 13.
3. ibid
4. Elizabeth Meyer et al, Incidence Trends of Type 1 and Type 2 Diabetes among Youths, 2002–2012 N Engl J Med 2017;376:1419-29.
5. Kirsten Bibbins-Domingo, Ph.D., M.D., Pamela Coxson, Ph.D., Mark J. Pletcher, M.D., M.P.H., James Lightwood, Ph.D., and Lee Goldman, M.D., M.P.H. Adolescent Overweight and Future Adult Coronary Heart Disease N Engl J Med 2007;357:2371-9
6. Kuczmarski RJ, Ogden CL, Guo SS, et al. 2000 CDC growth charts for the United States: Methods and development. National Center for Health Statistics. Vital Health Stat 11(246). 2002 Library of Congress Cataloging-in-Publication Data
7. ibid
8. The Five W's Of EDCs, viewed 28 January, 2018, https://endocrinenews.endocrine.org/wp-content/uploads/Hormone1114.pdf
9. Australian Guide to Healthy Eating, viewed 29 July 2017 https://www.eatforhealth.gov.au/guidelines/australian-guide-healthy-eating
10. The GBD 2015 Obesity Collaborators, Health Effects of Overweight and Obesity in 195 Countries over 25 Years, July 6, 2017, Vol. 377, No. 1, p. 1.
11. Dr George and Penny Blair-West, Food Loving Kids: Taste with your Face, 2010, p. 3.
12. Professor David Ludwig, Ending the Food Fight – Guide your child to a healthy weight in a fast food / fake food world, 2007, Houghton Mifflin.
13. Estruch R *et al* for PREDIMED Study Co-investigators. Primary prevention of cardiovascular disease with a Mediterranean diet. New Eng J Med 2013; 368:1279-1290. Harvard Health on the benefits of the Mediterranean diet https://www.health.harvard.edu/blog/a-practical-guide-to-the-mediterranean-diet-2019032116194
14. Nutrition Australia, viewed 30 July 2017, www.nutritionaustralia.org/national/resource/australian-dietary-guidelines-recommended-daily-intakes
15. Frederick F. Samaha, M.D., Nayyar Iqbal, M.D., Prakash Seshadri, M.D., Kathryn L. Chicano, C.R.N.P., Denise A. Daily, R.D., Joyce McGrory, C.R.N.P., Terrence Wil-liams, B.S., Monica Williams, Edward J. Gracely, Linda Stern, A Low-Carbohydrate as Compared with a Low-Fat Diet in Severe Obesity, N Engl J Med 2003; 348:2074-2081.
16. Stephen B. Sondike, Nancy Copperman, RD Marc, S. Jacobson, Effects of a low-carbohydrate diet on weight loss and cardiovascular risk factor in overweight adolescents, the Journal of Pediatrics
17. Estruch R *et al* for PREDIMED Study Co-investigators. Primary prevention of cardiovascular disease with a Mediterranean diet. New Eng J Med 2013; 368:1279-1290.

18 Saner C et al. Evidence for Protein Leverage in Children and Adolescents with Obesity. Obesity, published March 6 2020. https://onlinelibrary.wiley.com/doi/full/10.1002/oby.22755
19 Harvard Medical School, Healthy Eating: A guide to the new nutrition, page 17, March 2016
20 Harvard Medical School, Healthy Eating: A guide to the new nutrition, page 29, March 2016
21 Diet Doctor, viewed 30 July 2017, https:www.dietdoctor.com
22 (Eur J Epidemiol. 2018 Sep; 33(9):811-829. doi: 10.1007/s10654-018-0380-1. Epub 2018 Mar 28.
23 Levels of physical activity intensity, viewed 29 July 2017 http://www.healthyweight.health.gov.au
24 Australia's Physical Activity and Sedentary Behaviour Guidelines, viewed 29 July 2017, http://www.health.gov.au/internet/main/publishing.nsf/content/health-pubhlth-strateg-phys-act-guidelines#families
25 Jacob A. Nota, Meredith E. Coles. Shorter sleep duration and longer sleep onset latency are related to difficulty disengaging attention from negative emotional images in individuals with elevated transdiagnostic repetitive negative think-ing. Journal of Behavior Therapy and Experimental Psychiatry, 2018; 58: 114 DOI: 10.1016/j.jbtep.2017.10.003
26 Feinberg I, Campbell G Sleep EEG changes during adolescence: An index of a fundamental brain reorganization. Brain and Cognition Volume 72, Issue 1, 2010, 56-65.
27 Christakis NA and Fowler JH The spread of obesity in a large social network over 32 years. Neg J Med 2007. 357:370-379.
28 GBD 2015 Obesity Collaborators, Health Effects of Overweight and Obesity in 195 Countries over 25 Years, July 6, 2017, Vol. 377, No. 1, pp. 13–27.
29 Johann Hari, Lost Connections – Uncovering the Real Causes of Depression – and the Surprising Solutions, Bloomsbury, 2018
30 Roslyn Saunders, Emotional Sobriety: finding raw courage for recovery from co-dependence, 2017, page 44.
31 Professor George Chrousos, The concepts of stress and stress system disorders. Overview of physical and behavioral homeostasis, viewed 29 July, 2017 https://www.researchgate.net/profile/George_Chrousos/publication/21616289_The_concepts_of_stress_and_stress_system_disorders_Overview_of_physical_and_behavioral_homeostasis/links/00b7d520a3e93f1cf3000000.pdf
32 Creating a mind map, viewed 6 August 2017, https://imindmap.com/how-to-mind-map/
33 Brenda Goodman, Obesity Puts Young Kids at Risk of Social Isolation, WebMD, viewed 6 August, 2017, http://www.webmd.com/children/news/20110916/obesity-puts-young-kids-at-risk-of-social-isolation#1
34 Bruce Headeya, Ruud Muffelsb, and Gert G. Wagnerc, Long-running German pan-el survey shows that personal and economic choices, not just genes, matter for happiness, viewed 28, January 2017,PNAS,2007 http://www.pnas.org/content/pnas/107/42/17922.full.pdf

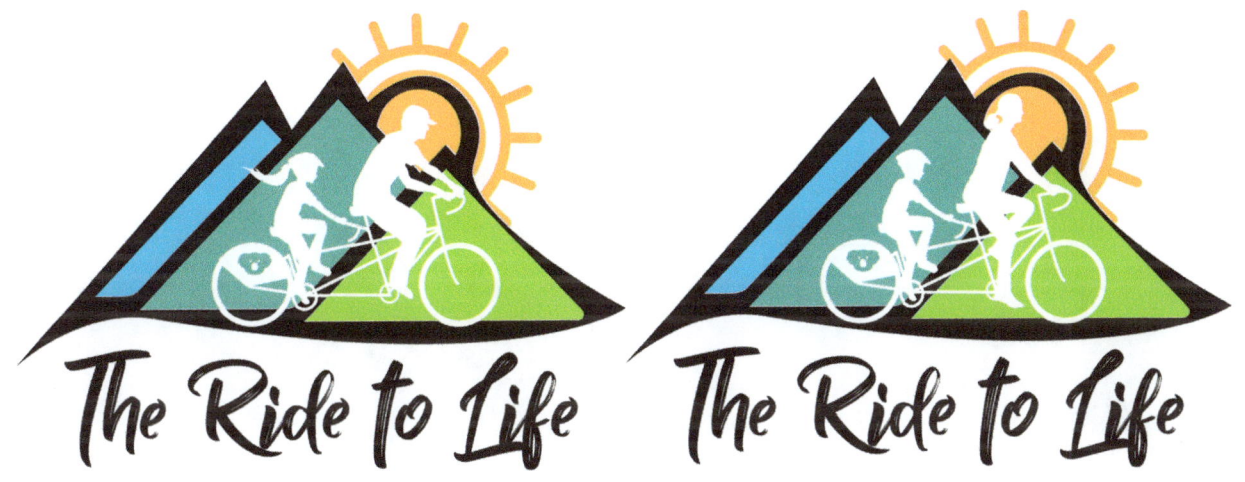

www.ingramcontent.com/pod-product-compliance
Lightning Source LLC
Chambersburg PA
CBHW061132010526
44107CB00068B/2916